Identified versus Statistical Lives

Population-Level Bioethics Series

Ethics and the Public's Health

Series Editors

Nir Eyal, Harvard Medical School

Daniel Wikler, Harvard School of Public Health

Editorial Board

Dan Brock, Harvard University

John Broome, Oxford University

Norman Daniels, Harvard University

Marc Fleurbaey, Princeton University

Julio Frenk, Harvard University

Frances Kamm, Harvard University

Daniel Hausman, University of Wisconsin-Madison

Michael Marmot, University College, London

Christopher Murray, Institute for Health Metrics and Evaluation, University of Washington

Amartya Sen, Harvard University

Volumes in the Series

Inequalities in Health
Concepts, Measures, and Ethics
Edited by Nir Eyal, Samia A. Hurst, Ole F. Norheim, and Dan Wikler

Identified versus Statistical Lives
An Interdisciplinary Perspective
Edited by I. Glenn Cohen, Norman Daniels, and Nir Eyal

Identified versus Statistical Lives

AN INTERDISCIPLINARY PERSPECTIVE

Edited by I. Glenn Cohen
Norman Daniels
and
Nir Eyal

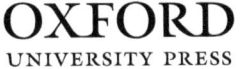

OXFORD
UNIVERSITY PRESS

Oxford University Press is a department of the University of
Oxford. It furthers the University's objective of excellence in research,
scholarship, and education by publishing worldwide.

Oxford   New York
Auckland   Cape Town   Dar es Salaam   Hong Kong   Karachi
Kuala Lumpur   Madrid   Melbourne   Mexico City   Nairobi
New Delhi   Shanghai   Taipei   Toronto

With offices in
Argentina   Austria   Brazil   Chile   Czech Republic   France   Greece
Guatemala   Hungary   Italy   Japan   Poland   Portugal   Singapore
South Korea   Switzerland   Thailand   Turkey   Ukraine   Vietnam

Oxford is a registered trademark of Oxford University Press
in the UK and certain other countries.

Published in the United States of America by
Oxford University Press
198 Madison Avenue, New York, NY 10016

© Oxford University Press 2015

All rights reserved. No part of this publication may be reproduced, stored in
a retrieval system, or transmitted, in any form or by any means, without the prior
permission in writing of Oxford University Press, or as expressly permitted by law,
by license, or under terms agreed with the appropriate reproduction rights organization.
Inquiries concerning reproduction outside the scope of the above should be sent to the
Rights Department, Oxford University Press, at the address above.

You must not circulate this work in any other form
and you must impose this same condition on any acquirer.

Library of Congress Cataloging-in-Publication Data
Identified versus statistical lives : an interdisciplinary perspective/edited by I. Glenn Cohen,
Norman Daniels, and Nir Eyal.
   p. ; cm.
Includes bibliographical references.
ISBN 978–0–19–021747–1 (hardcover : alk. paper)
I. Cohen, I. Glenn, editor.   II. Daniels, Norman, 1942–, editor.   III. Eyal, Nir M. (Nir Mordechay),
1970–, editor.
[DNLM: 1. Health Care Rationing-ethics. 2. Empathy. 3. Health Policy. WA 525]
RA410.5
362.1—dc23

9780190217471

For Dan Brock

CONTENTS

Acknowledgments ix
Contributors xi

Statistical versus Identified Persons: An Introduction 1
GLENN COHEN, NORMAN DANIELS, AND NIR EYAL

PART I } Social Science

1. On the Psychology of the Identifiable Victim Effect 13
   DEBORAH A. SMALL

2. "Dual-Process" Models of the Mind and the "Indentifiable Victim Effect" 24
   PETER RAILTON

PART II } Ethics and Political Philosophy

3. Identified versus Statistical Lives: Some Introductory Issues and Arguments 43
   DAN W. BROCK

4. Welfarism, Equity, and the Choice between Statistical and Identified Victims 53
   MATTHEW D. ADLER

5. Risking Life and Limb: How to Discount Harms by Their Improbability 77
   MICHAEL OTSUKA

6. Concentrated Risk, the Coventry Blitz, Chamberlain's Cancer 94
   NIR EYAL

7. Can There be Moral Force to Favoring an Identified over a Statistical Life? 110
   NORMAN DANIELS

8. Statistical People and Counterfactual Indeterminacy 124
   CASPAR HARE

9. How (Not) to Argue for the Rule of Rescue: Claims of Individuals versus Group Solidarity   137
MARCEL VERWEIJ

10. Why Not Empathy?   150
MICHAEL SLOTE

PART III } **Applications**

11. Identified versus Statistical Lives in US Civil Litigation: Of Standing, Ripeness, and Class Actions   161
I. GLENN COHEN

12. Statistical Lives in Environmental Law   174
LISA HEINZERLING

13. Treatment versus Prevention in the Fight against HIV/AIDS and the Problem of Identified versus Statistical Lives   182
JOHANN FRICK

14. From Biology to Policy: Ethical and Economic Issues in HIV Treatment-as-Prevention   203
TILL BÄRNIGHAUSEN AND MAX ESSEX

15. Testing, Treating, and Trusting   213
JONATHAN WOLFF

Index 219

ACKNOWLEDGMENTS

This book came out of the Harvard University Program in Ethics and Health 2012 annual conference. The editors would like to thank Harvard University's Program in Ethics and Health, the Harvard Global Health Institute, the Petrie-Flom Center for Health Law Policy, Biotechnology, and Bioethics at Harvard Law School, the Oswald DeN. Cammann Fund, and the Edward J. Safra Center for Ethics, for cosponsoring that conference. They would also like to thank Kathy Paras, Jeannette Austin, Glaudine Mtshali, and Francesca Holinko for their help in running that conference, and Stephen Resch for helping us to conceive it. The editors are also grateful to the Otto and Marie Neurath Isotype Collection at the University of Reading, and to Rob Banham, Diane Billbey, and the graphic design society RU-CMYK (especially Craig Melvin and Emma Saunders) for help in accessing their archive from which the cover art for this book was taken. Carol Maglitta made wonderful designs for this volume and the series. Kaitlin Burroughs provided outstanding assistance with the editing and formatting of the book and Richard Isomaki ran a swift and effective line edit on the entire volume. Harvard's Global Health Institute provided generous financial support for further work on this volume. Glenn Cohen thanks the Radcliffe Institute for Advanced Studies and the Greenwall Foundation Faculty Scholarship in Bioethics, which funded the year he used to work on this project. The editors are grateful for permission to reprint Caspar Hare's chapter, originally published as "Obligations to Merely Statistical People" in *Journal of Philosophy* 109, nos. 5–6, June 2012.

I. Glenn Cohen
Norman Daniels
Nir Eyal

CONTRIBUTORS

Matthew D. Adler is Richard A. Horvitz Professor of Law and Professor of Economics, Philosophy and Public Policy at Duke University.

Till Bärnighausen is Associate Professor of Global Health in the Department of Global Health and Population, Harvard School of Public Health and Senior Epidemiologist, Africa Centre, University of KwaZulu Natal.

Dan W. Brock is Frances Glessner Lee Professor of Medical Ethics, Emeritus in the Department of Global Health and Social Medicine, Harvard Medical School.

I. Glenn Cohen is Professor, Harvard Law School and Director, Petrie-Flom Center for Health Law Policy, Biotechnology, and Bioethics.

Norman Daniels is Mary B. Saltonstall Professor of Population Ethics and Professor of Ethics and Population Health, Harvard School of Public Health.

Max Essex is Mary Woodard Lasker Professor of Health Sciences in the Department of Immunology and Infectious Diseases, Harvard School of Public Health.

Nir Eyal is Associate Professor of Global Health and Social Medicine (Bioethics), Harvard Medical School and Associate Professor of Global Health and Population, Harvard TH Chan School of Public Health.

Johann Frick is Assistant Professor in the Department of Philosophy and the Center for Human Values, Princeton University.

Caspar Hare is Associate Professor of Philosophy in the Department of Linguistics and Philosophy at MIT.

Lisa Heinzerling is Justice William J. Brennan, Jr. Professor of Law, Georgetown University Law Center and formerly Associate Administrator, Office of Policy, US Environmental Protection Agency.

Michael Otsuka is Professor of Philosophy, London School of Economics.

Peter Railton is Kavka Distinguished University Professor, Department of Philosophy at the University of Michigan.

Michael Slote is UST Professor of Ethics, Department of Philosophy, University of Miami.

Deborah A. Small is Associate Professor of Marketing at the Wharton School, with a secondary appointment in Psychology, University of Pennsylvania.

Marcel Verweij is Chair of Philosophy, Department of Social Sciences, Wageningen University, The Netherlands.

Jonathan Wolff is Dean of Arts & Humanities and Professor of Philosophy at University College London.

Statistical versus Identified Persons: An Introduction

I. Glenn Cohen, Norman Daniels, and Nir Eyal

On August 5, 2010, a cave-in left 33 miners trapped nearly half a mile underground in a copper and gold mine near the small Chilean city of Copiapó. The Chilean government embarked on a massive rescue effort, with assistance from multiple international teams, experts, and donors. For weeks, the men's personal stories were featured on TV screens all around the world. After 69 days, on October 13, 2010, the trapped miners finally ascended, to an international sigh of relief. Speaking upon the completion of the rescue, Chilean president Sebastian Pinera estimated that the complicated mission cost US$10–20 million. However, he added, "Every peso was well spent" (CNN Wire Staff 2010; Epatko 2010).

There is a puzzle here. Many mine safety measures that would have been more cost-effective, and many unrelated more cost-effective interventions for health, had not been taken in Chile earlier, either by the Chilean government or by international donors. Why did we suddenly witness a Chilean and worldwide special will to rescue these 33 men?

The Chilean story is a vivid, real illustration of a problem that Thomas Schelling (1968) first identified as the problem of identified versus statistical lives; a short time later, Charles Fried (1969) wrote a seminal article about that problem. Albert Jonsen (1986) identified a related issue, the so-called rule of rescue, which others have characterized in medical settings as "the powerful human proclivity to rescue a single identified endangered life, regardless of cost, at the expense of many nameless faces who will therefore be denied health care" (Osborne and Evans 1994, 779). We shall refer to the puzzling phenomenon, approached from different angles by Schelling, Fried, and Jonsen, as

> *The identified person bias*: A greater inclination to assist (and avoid harming) persons and groups identified as those at high risk of great

harm than to assist (and avoid harming) persons and groups who will suffer (or already suffer) similar harm but are not identified (as yet).

Although the word "bias" often takes on a normative hue, our usage is merely descriptive. We do not mean "bias" in a pejorative sense that assumes lack of justification. Indeed, much of this volume addresses the question whether the identified person bias is justified.

The bias toward assisting identified persons has many expressions both in health care and in other domains. Many nations fund expensive intensive care and dialysis for people who otherwise are at high risk of dying soon. They do so even though many preventative interventions would avert more deaths per dollar, often from the same diseases. Is that a mistake? In particular, should poor and middle-income countries never fund expensive dialysis so long as they lack the funds for more cost-effective interventions for most everyone in need, including medication for high blood pressure (a cause of kidney failure and the need for dialysis)? In rich countries, there is active debate on funding particularly expensive drugs that are the last line of defense against cancer. One contemporary example is Ipilimumab, prescribed for previously treated advanced melanoma. In the United Kingdom, when used for that indication, Ipilimumab costs £42,200 per quality-adjusted life year (QALY) gained (NICE 2012, 26)—more than allowed in previous funding thresholds. Should the United Kingdom instead let advanced cancer patients die and focus on cost-effective interventions to prevent (advanced) cancer and other diseases? If this case shows bias in favor of identified cancer patients, is the bias justified?

Examples of the identified person bias abound outside health care as well. Fundraisers for charities know that telling a story about a specific person in need is more likely to produce a donation than citing statistics about many people in comparable need. Are fundraisers here exploiting what should be seen as irrationality on our part? In tort law and environmental policy, should a tortfeasor be held more liable when it does a reckless or negligent action that harms a particular identified person as opposed to putting an as yet unidentified individual at comparable risk? How should we evaluate the costs associated with the National Ambient Air Quality Standards of the Clean Air Act, which regulates air pollution levels in the United States, cost that are currently justified as protecting statistical and not identified persons?

Is the identified person bias one big mistake on our part—a "bias" in the pejorative sense? It is easy to dismiss an absolutist rule of rescue that gives an implausible lexical (that is, absolute) priority to people and populations identified as high-risk. For example, America's Medicare refuses to even consider the opportunity cost when assessing whether to fund death-postponing drugs like Ipilimumab—which commentators have found unwise (Brock 2006). It is also easy to see that we are not doing enough on hypertension and cancer prevention, on infectious disease prevention, on the social determinants of health, and on other cost-effective measures that would prevent death and disability for many more statistical persons than rescue interventions would.

But the fundamental ethical question about the identified person bias remains real. A genuine question persists as to whether we should give some priority to identified persons over statistical ones. Failing to prioritize identified persons seems under some circumstances ethically wrong to most people, even after careful reflection. We conjecture that many people would reject the suggestion that poor countries should not provide life-saving and highly cost-effective surgeries such as relatively simple congenital heart surgeries (at levels 1 or 2 of surgical complication), which move a child from a nearly certain death to a pretty certain life with no follow-up, until they have funded all the even more cost-effective prophylactic interventions they can fund. Should that strong intuition be rejected?

This volume asks three questions about the identified person bias:

1. When precisely does the identified person bias arise? And what exactly does it consist in? For example, is it simply a matter of a very human response to the vivid human faces of people with personal stories, in the hospital ward or on TV screens? Is it something that arises only when the risks are known, only under strict uncertainty, or regardless of how much we can specify the risk? Does that bias arise only when few victims are involved? (Stalin, it is claimed, memorably said, "The death of one man is a tragedy, the death of millions is a statistic.") And when we are inclined to prioritize identified persons, are we just inclined to help them, or typically also inclined to feel in certain ways (say, compassionately) and to suppress thought about certain things (say, potentially relevant considerations such as cost to others and to society, health and welfare distribution in previous decades, personal desert, and personal responsibility)?

2. What, if anything, might justify giving priority to identified persons at risk? After all, they are not necessarily poorer or sicker over their entire lives than the rest of us, or otherwise necessarily worse off in their personal outcomes. Priority to identified persons does not necessarily assist the deserving, or the near and dear, or whomever else we may think we should prioritize. *Ex hypothesi*, focus on those at highest risk does not ensure that more lives or QALYs are saved; on the contrary, it often ensures that fewer are saved. Nor is this necessarily the familiar question about "aggregation" (whether preventing tiny harms to scores of people can ever be more urgent than preventing a momentous harm to one). Risk does not always translate into harm. So is our inclination to prioritize identified persons warranted, and (if so) on what ground?

3. What would be the practical implications for law, public health, medicine, and the environment of accepting the priority given to identified persons, or of forsaking it—if we could successfully do so? For example, is it appropriate that in some ways tort law requires an identified victim to bring forth suits? Can our moral position on the bias help us decide how to allocate resources between HIV/AIDS treatment and prevention in the developing world, and evaluate so-called "treatment-as-prevention"?

The book brings together behavioral psychologists, ethicists, epidemiologists, and legal experts to address all three questions. The first part of the book further characterizes the identified person bias; the second debates the ethical justification of that bias; and the third turns to practical applications.

Part I: Social Science

Part I of the book examines the existing social and evolutionary accounts of the identified person bias—the data that support it and what exactly those data show.

In her chapter "On the Psychology of the Identifiable Victim Effect," Deborah A. Small reviews the social psychology experiments that demonstrate the identified person bias in the lab and in the field. She asks what manipulations make the bias manifest. As she shows, early anecdotal evidence for an identified person bias could not distinguish the effect of identifiability from that of sympathy; that is, one used to be unable to tell whether any emotional reaction is caused by the victim's status as "identifiable" or by the particular information by which the victim was made identifiable. Studies that Small coauthored and that her chapter reviews show that making someone identifiable even in the crudest sense—for example, merely identifying a person with an anonymous number—has significant impact on the generosity and behavior of subjects toward that person. Small then grounds the explanation for these kinds of effects in two psychological mechanisms, dual processing and psychological distancing. She shows that reducing psychological distance to anonymous victims can facilitate caring.

Peter Railton's chapter, " 'Dual-Process' Models of the Mind and the 'Statistical Victim Effect,' " continues this discussion of psychological mechanisms that might explain the favoring of identified persons over merely statistical ones. It also offers a normative analysis of how we should respond to such explanations. Building on the dual-process models that Small discusses, Railton asks what we can learn from studies of nonhuman animals and suggests that some roots of the identified person bias phenomenon may lie in elements of our brains that we share with animals. He argues that instead of understanding the identified person bias as "a conflict between Reason (System 2) and Passion (System 1)," we should "come to see System

1 (the affective system) as designed for experience-based construction of expectation-based evaluative models of situations, actions, and outcomes." He then explores what this account of the bias would mean for normative evaluation of it.

Part II: Ethics and Political Philosophy

Part II examines philosophical arguments in favor of and against the identified person bias. It is divided between authors who argue that there is little or no normative reason to prioritize identified persons over statistical ones, and ones who find substantial reasons to do so.

In the first camp, authors who find little or no reason to favor identified lives, are Dan W. Brock, Matthew Adler, Michael Otsuka, and Nir Eyal.

In "Identified vs. Statistical Lives: Some Introductory Issues and Arguments," Dan Brock reviews seven arguments that are commonly offered to establish that identified lives have greater intrinsic moral value than statistical lives: the rule of rescue, urgency, aggregation, priority to the worst off, uncertainty, temporal discounting, and special relationships. He argues that we should reject all of these arguments. The arguments sometimes (but not always) map onto distinctions that themselves are morally relevant, such as the distinction between the worse off and the better off. Sometimes they map onto psychologically salient but morally irrelevant distinctions. Brock then examines whether other forms of argument for the identified person might justify the bias. In his view, some arguments might actually depend on "the empirical claim that giving greater priority to identified lives in the specified circumstances either enables the saving of more lives, or produces more overall value." His conclusion is that "when, but only when, a morally important principle like priority to the worse off maps onto the identified/statistical difference, then the identified/statistical difference is morally important—but that is because of the other principle—in this case, priority to the worse off—not the difference between identified and statistical lives."

In "Welfarism, Equity, and the Choice between Statistical and Identified Victims," Matthew Adler examines whether welfarist theories in ethics—theories that morally evaluate choices only in light of the associated distributions of individual well-being—must reject any favoritism for identified over statistical lives. He provides an argument to show that "the problem of statistical versus identified lives cannot be settled at the level of welfarism, nor as part of the debate about CBA [cost-benefit analysis], nor even by rejecting utilitarianism. Ex ante and ex post equity-regarding approaches concur in embracing welfarism, rejecting CBA, and embracing a concern for an equitable distribution of well-being (thus rejecting utilitarianism). Their disagreement concerns a much more subtle problem: equity-regarding policy choice under conditions of uncertainty." Adler concludes that the problem of statistical versus identified lives is intimately connected to the ex ante/ex post debate and that the "welfarist who cares about equity must, further, decide whether the 'currency' for fair distribution is expected well-being (the ex ante approach) or final utilities (the ex post approach)."

Michael Otsuka's chapter, "Risking Life and Limb: How to Discount Harms by Their Improbability," examines the interplay between identifiability, probability, aggregation, and claims to assistance through ingenious thought experiments. Following Matthew Adler and others, Otsuka distinguishes what he calls "epistemic probabilities" defined as "frequencies relative to classes of events and persons about which statistical data is actually available" from what he calls "objective probabilities," namely "frequencies relative to classes of events and persons . . . that [in fact] share all the [same] causally relevant features—not merely the features about which good statistical data is actually available." Otsuka uses this distinction to set up a series of thought experiments that differ according to whether those facing disproportional risk do so in terms of epistemic probabilities or objective probabilities. He rejects the claim that mere statistical persons only have as much "claim" to assistance as does an "indeterminate person along the lines of a fictional character." Otsuka proposes that "we discount a complaint against suffering harm by the chance that *someone* would actually suffer such harm." That is distinct from "the more familiar proposal that we discount a person's complaint against suffering harm by the chance that *he* would suffer such harm."

In his chapter, "Concentrated Risk, the Coventry Blitz, Chamberlain's Cancer," Nir Eyal invokes historical events from the Battle of Britain to make a philosophical point. Eyal argues that while there may be contingent, instrumental, and derivative reasons to prioritize persons identified as facing concentrated risk (such as the danger that people will falsely perceive nonintervention as unfair and as expressive of disrespect), such reasons are not essential to allocation between identified and statistical persons. In particular, being identified as high-risk does not strengthen a person's inherent moral claims to protection, on either a subjective or an objective interpretation of risk. Fairness toward the worse off matters, but a person identified as high-risk is not necessarily worse off.

Others in the volume—Norman Daniels, Caspar Hare, Marcel Verweij, and Michael Slote—emphasize in their chapters reasons to vindicate our bias in favor of the identified person, and Johann Frick's applied chapter in Part III also takes a similar position.

In "Can There be Moral Force to Favoring an Identified over a Statistical Life?" Norman Daniels partially dissents from those who would treat the favoring of identified lives as a bias to be corrected and argues that "a case can be made for ascribing some normative force to the disposition, at least in certain circumstances." Specifically, if identified victims face greater risks than statistical ones, then the former count as worse off than those statistically at some risk, and justifiably in need of more assistance. Since both consequentialist and nonconsequentialist moral theories leave room for "reasonable disagreement" on the question whether to prioritize who are identified as high-risk over mere statistical victims, "public policy requires a form of procedural justice, specifically, a fair, deliberative process in which conflicting views are considered and rationales are developed for policies that rest on the most acceptable rationales."

Reacting in part to Daniels's work, Caspar Hare assesses the call of "merely statistical people" in his chapter, "Statistical People and Counterfactual Indeterminacy." He uses a series of thought experiments to generate two person-affecting antiaggregationist principles: (1) *Distribute bad effects*: Given a choice between doing something very good for one person but very bad for one person, and doing something very good for one person but quite bad for each of four people, you ought, other things being equal, to do the latter. (2) *Concentrate good effects*: Other things being equal, given a choice between doing something very good for one person and very bad for one person, and doing something quite good for four people and very bad for one person, you ought, other things being equal, to do the former. Hare suggests that together these principles "tell us that, other things being equal, you ought to save 'identified' rather than 'merely statistical' people in the cases we have looked at." He adds, however, that because the principles supporting these considerations "do not tell us how much those considerations matter," we should not give much consideration in favor of identified lives.

Marcel Verweij's chapter, "How (Not) to Argue for the Rule of Rescue: Claims of Individuals versus Group Solidarity," makes two central claims: that individualist approaches to ethics will not succeed in justifying an identified person bias and, second, that collectivist approaches might. As to the first claim, he suggests that contractualist approaches to ethics, like those championed by Tim Scanlon, which focus on what we owe individuals, can only justify favoring persons identified as being at high risk and in need of rescue if they adopt an ex ante perspective that focuses on large risks to individuals, not on large harms to them. But their moral complaints, he argues, will be clearly outweighed from a consistent contractualist perspective by the complaints of people who will die if they are not rescued. Excluding ex post perspectives cannot be justified. So for Verweij, Scanlon's contractualism cannot justify the rule of rescue. Verweij sees a more promising argument in favor of priority to identified persons, namely "the importance of the fact that people are standing together, sharing hope and fear, and supporting each other in the face of—and fight against—disaster." He associates the latter idea with a more collectivist solidarity and argues that in some instances it can be action-guiding. However, he cautions that the value of solidarity has to be balanced against other values, like that of saving lives, and that the importance that solidarity will play in these analyses is proportional to how much the community as such is under threat from neglect of identified persons.

In "Why Not Empathy?" Michael Slote registers a dissent from what he sees as the consequentialist or rationalist and intuitionist thrust of the other contributions to this volume, which fail to take seriously the moral importance of emotions. Building on his earlier work on moral sentimentalism, he develops an emotion-centered virtue ethics approach to the identified persons question. A foundational view that he ascribes to Peter Singer, among others, rejects partiality as a basis for moral decision-making. For Slote, "empathy is not only partial but also a basic ingredient in our moral concepts. Our moral thinking correlates with differences in empathy insofar as we think that what goes more against empathy is also morally worse." Indeed, according to Slote, "moral goodness is identical with having full and fully empathic concern for others and the wrongness of an action approach consists in its reflecting or exhibiting a lack of such concern for others." Applying this conclusion to our context, he argues, justifies favoring identified persons in some circumstances, as a matter of empathy.

Part III: Applications

The final part of this book turns from theory to practice. It examines several areas of law, medicine, and public health where the phenomenon of bias may have serious effects on public policy.

I. Glenn Cohen's chapter, "Identified versus Statistical Lives in US Civil Litigation: Of Standing, Ripeness, and Class Actions," examines how the identified person bias manifests itself in US federal civil litigation. First, he argues that two doctrines employed by courts to help determine whether a controversy can be heard at the present moment—the standing of individual plaintiffs and the ripeness of the dispute—press litigants to bring claims on behalf of identified and not statistical victims and will cause courts to dismiss cases in which the injury envisioned will affect primarily statistical persons. Second, he discusses the way one modern innovation of American civil procedure, the class action device, acts as a partial salve that allows for the adjudication of harms to statistical victims through the litigation of a representative identified claimant, or a "representative life": a middle concept between identified and statistical lives where an identified life stands in for a much larger number of (as yet) statistical lives.

"Statistical Lives in Environmental Law," Lisa Heinzerling's contribution to this volume, shifts the focus from civil litigation in general to environmental disputes in particular. Heinzerling argues that "it is barely an exaggeration to say there are no identified lives in environmental law," and indeed "as it relates to human health, environmental law is arguably defined by reference to the protection of statistical, not identified, lives." Indeed, so strong is the connection between environmental law and statistical lives, she writes, that the legal corpus often seems "disinclined to think of identified victims as environmental casualties." Given the well-known biases against statistical lives that are emphasized elsewhere in this volume, one might therefore "expect environmental law to offer relatively weak protections for human health." She shows, however, that quite the opposite is true, and that major US environmental laws provide exceedingly strong protections for human health despite their purported focus on statistical lives. Heinzerling substantiates this claim by drawing on a myriad of examples from environmental law, from ambient air quality standards to pesticides.

In " 'Treatment' versus 'Prevention' in the Fight against HIV/AIDS and the Problem of Identified versus Statistical Lives," Johann Frick tackles a long-standing dispute among researchers and policymakers involved in battling the HIV/AIDS pandemic. That dispute pits proponents of scaling up antiretroviral treatment for people already suffering from AIDS against advocates for a focus on allegedly more cost-effective prevention measures. Frick challenges a central premise of some of the latter advocates: that if one believes that all human lives have equal worth, there can be no sound moral basis for giving any priority to the saving of identified over statistical lives, all else equal. Like Daniels, he argues that the greater risk facing some identified lives matters morally, other things being equal. Frick shows this through several thought experiments. He adds, however, that it matters whether decisions on policy happen before or after some are identified as high-risk. Frick concludes that the problem in the case of HIV/AIDS is crucially different from some other identified versus statistical lives policy choices: "Because it is an ongoing problem, our decision is never taken from a point of view that is ex ante for everyone."

Till Bärnighausen and Max Essex's chapter, "From Biology to Policy: Ethical and Economic Issues in HIV Treatment-as-Prevention," shifts the focus from the choice between treatment and prevention to what in public health has become known as treatment-as-prevention. The latter is a public health technique that puts HIV-positive persons on antiretroviral therapy upon HIV diagnosis and regardless of white blood cell count, partly in order to decrease the chance of HIV transmission to others. In essence, individuals start therapy earlier than the most (cost) effective timing for their own health, as a preventative: in order to help reduce infection of others. The authors review the evidence from existing studies on this promising intervention, including a large study conducted by one of them. They then imagine a world where it has been firmly established that treatment-as-prevention can significantly reduce HIV incidence in general populations affected by the HIV epidemic. They lay out new ethical and economic challenges that will present themselves once treatment-as-prevention has been identified as effective in generalized HIV epidemics. Different perspectives on the identified victim bias might inflect public policy choices as to treatment-as-prevention.

Jonathan Wolff in "Testing, Treating, and Trusting," expresses skepticism that clinicians and policymakers in developing countries can conform to "maximization" arguments for cost-effective preventive measures for HIV/AIDS instead of treating people who have been infected. But he also cautions that if treating leads to more risky sexual behaviors, then we face an assurance problem that adds to the difficulty of getting everyone tested, in contexts where HIV stigma is significant. "Test and treat" (roughly, an earlier name for "treatment-as-prevention") faces compliance challenges on both the "test" and the "treat" components of the approach.

We hope that the various contributions to this book will help readers learn about the identified person bias, its cognitive underpinnings, its justifiability or lack thereof, and its practical import.

References

Brock, Dan W. 2006. "How Much Is More Life Worth?" *Hastings Center Report* 36 (3): 17–19.
CNN Wire Staff. 2010. "After a Final Day Together, Miners Begin to Disband." CNN, October 15.
Epatko, Larisa. 2010. "Chile's Mine Rescue: Costs and Benefits." *PBS Newshour*.
Fried, Charles. "Value of Life." 1969. *Harvard Law Review* 82 (7): 1415–37.
Jonsen, Albert R. 1986. "Bentham in a Box: Technology Assessment and Health Care Allocation." *Journal of Law, Medicine & Ethics* 14 (3–4): 172–74.
NICE. 2012. TA268: Ipilimumab for Previously Treated Advanced (Unresectable or Metastatic) Melanoma. December 12 (cited July 2, 2013). Available from http://www.nice.org.uk/nicemedia/live/14001/61847/61847.pdf.
Osborne, M., and T. W. Evans. 1994. "Allocation of Resources in Intensive Care: A Transatlantic Perspective." *Lancet* 343 (8900): 778–80.
Schelling, Thomas. 1968. "The Life You Save May Be Your Own." In *Problems in Public Expenditure Analysis*, edited by Samuel B. Chase, 127–62. Washington, DC: Brookings Institution.

PART } I

Social Science

1 }

On the Psychology of the Identifiable Victim Effect

Deborah A. Small

When do people respond to others' misfortunes? How come certain disasters and victims attract a lot of attention from the media and others attract next to none? How are scarce resources allocated when needs are pervasive? Do people follow a utilitarian principle and allocate money efficiently—where it can do the most good? Or does human psychology follow its own rules that diverge from efficiency?

Recent large-scale disasters provide tests of the public's sympathy and its ability to make good decisions. Following the earthquakes in Haiti (2010) and Japan (2011), people around the world appeared impressively big-hearted by pledging an estimated $4.6 billion to Haiti and $4.95 billion to Japan. The public has also demonstrated extraordinary compassion in responses to certain ill-fated individuals, such as Natalee Holloway or JonBenet Ramsey, whose victimhood became media sensations. Moreover, certain individual victims have even served as the rationale behind legislation. For example, former press secretary James Brady, who was shot during the attempted assassination of President Ronald Reagan, served as the impetus for the Brady Handgun Violence Prevention Act in 1993. Similarly, after the Casey Anthony trial, in which Anthony did not report that her daughter, Caylee, had been missing for a month, a number of bills, commonly referred to as "Caylee's Law," were introduced.

In contrast to these examples of compassionate public responses, there are widespread and persistent misfortunes and needs close to home and around the world (such as poverty and water- and insect-borne disease) that fail to arouse sympathy and suitable collective action. For every Natalee Holloway, there are millions of individuals whose faces are hidden and whose tragic stories are never told.

These examples demonstrate a phenomenon referred to as the identifiable victim effect, the subject of this volume. The effect was first discussed as such by Thomas Schelling (1968) and refers to the psychological tendency to disproportionately concentrate resources on specific, identifiable victims relative to statistical victims. Countless anecdotes of kidnap victims provide a rich intuition for the effect. This intuition has been supplemented and clarified by a great body of empirical research both in the laboratory and in the field, which provide a deeper understanding of the psychological mechanisms driving the effect.

The purpose of this chapter is to answer the questions presented at the beginning of the chapter through a review of descriptive psychological research on aid allocation decisions. The chapter does not seek to resolve the normative question of how scarce resources should be allocated. Instead normative theory—in particular utilitarianism (Bentham [1843] 1948; Mill [1863] 1906)—provides a useful benchmark to which actual decisions can be contrasted. While the value of this normative model is debated elsewhere in this volume, it is the predominant normative benchmark in economics and decision theory. Thus, in contrast to this standard for which all lives are valued equally and scarce resources are allocated in ways that maximize impact, this chapter describes how people actually make such decisions.

1. Empirical Evidence in the Lab and Field

Early work on the identifiable victim effect seemed to imply that it was part of a more general effect of reference group size. Specifically, research on psychophysical numbing suggests that people are sensitive to proportions rather than absolute numbers of lives (Featherstonhaugh et al. 1997; Jenni and Loewenstein 1997). For example, an event that causes 10 deaths within a very small community of 200 tends to evoke a great amount of concern, as 10 out of 200 is a fairly large proportion. Yet people exhibit much less concern if that same event causes 10 deaths throughout a large population of millions of people. Ten deaths out of many million is merely a "drop in the bucket." An identifiable victim becomes her own reference group—one out of one. This maximum proportion can partly explain why identifiable victims receive disproportionate support. Yet this reference group effect does not tell the whole story.

A great deal of research in the past 10 years demonstrates that beyond a simple reference group explanation, there is something special about being identifiable. To begin, empirical isolation of an identifiable victim effect was particularly important because the anecdotal contrast of a specific victim and victim statistics is confounded by a variety of informative factors. Specifically, each anecdote of an identifiable victim contains its own unique story and image. As stories and images can evoke sympathy, it is possible that they are the true cause of sympathy, rather than the victim's status as "identifiable." In any particular case, one cannot know what fosters the emotional reaction and behavioral response. Is it the victim's status as "identifiable," or is the particular information (i.e., story and imagery) by which he or she was made identifiable? This makes it critical to tease apart identifiability from the information by which someone becomes identifiable.

Small and Loewenstein (2003) conducted controlled experiments to rule out information confounds. In one study, they gave each member of a group of participants $10 and a number. Based on a random drawing, half the participants (the "victims") were made to return the money to the experimenter. Next, the other half of participants—those who kept their $10—had the opportunity to share some of it with a "victim" in a setup based on an anonymous allocation task called the "dictator game" from experimental economics. In the identifiable victim condition, the potential giver first drew the number of the victim from the bag, and then decided how to give to that victim (knowing that he or she would never learn the actual identity of the victim). In the unidentifiable condition, the potential giver decided how much to give immediately before drawing the victim's number. Allocations were about twice as large, on average, in the identifiable condition than in the unidentifiable condition, despite the fact that the experimental manipulation contained no meaningful information (name, picture, etc.) about the victim. That is, merely identifying a person with an anonymous number was sufficient to increase generosity. A separate study found similar results when participants rated how sympathetic they felt toward the person whose number they had drawn or were about to draw (see Loewenstein and Small 2007). This finding was replicated in another study by Small and Loewenstein (2003), in which donations to a Habitat for Humanity home were solicited in the field. Here identifiability was manipulated by informing respondents that the family who would attain the home either "has been selected" or "will be selected." In neither condition were respondents told which family had been or would be selected; the only difference between conditions was in whether the decision had already been made. When the family had been identified but remained anonymous, contributions to the charity were significantly greater.

Building on these early findings, Kogut and Ritov (2005a) demonstrated that a single identifiable victim receives more support than a group of identifiable victims. In several studies, participants were asked to contribute to a costly life-saving treatment needed by either one or eight sick children. The total amount of money needed was held constant regardless of the number of children it would help. When the victims were described with minimal detail (age, name, picture), and when participants were only faced with the option of donating either to one or to eight children, contributions to one child exceeded contributions to eight children. Yet when the same numbers of victims were described without any identifying information, the number of victims had no effect. In other words, the combination of identification and singularity (i.e., one beneficiary) elicited extraordinary sympathy. Finally, when a separate set of participants were asked to choose between contributing to one or eight victims, most chose to donate to the group of eight even if they were made identifiable (Kogut and Ritov 2005b). That is, laypeople buy into the social utility maximizing option (i.e., recognize that it is better to help more people) when the number of victims is salient and comparable. However, when the comparison is not there, they respond based on their sympathy, which is inverse to the magnitude of total need in the group (see also Hsee and Rottenstreich 2004).

More recently, observational field data revealed a similar pattern. Galak, Small, and Stephen (2011) examined data from Kiva.org, the leading micro-lending intermediary whose mission is to alleviate poverty through microfinance. This organization permits borrowers, who do not have access to traditional forms of credit, to submit proposals for small uncollateralized loans for their entrepreneurial endeavors. Proposals typically consist of a description of the borrower and his or her business and a picture. Lenders review proposals online and make interest-free loans with the intent of helping a borrower grow the business. Critical to the study of identifiable victims, borrowers can be single individuals or can borrow in groups. Historically, loans to groups have had higher repayment rates due to peer screening (Varian 1990), and peer monitoring (Stiglitz 1990), which makes them more financially viable (Yunus 1999). Yet consistent with Kogut and Ritov (2005b), the data reveal that people prefer lending to individuals and that lending goes down as the group size of the borrower increases.

To summarize, empirical research on the identifiable victim effect has sought to disentangle identifiability from the information about an identified victim or to control for it. Research has found that people behave more generously toward an identifiable victim than to an unidentified one. Subsequent research demonstrated the remarkable power of the number one, or in this case, one victim. As the number of identifiable victims increases, generosity declines. In the next section, I discuss evidence about the psychological process driving the identifiable victim effect.

2. On the Psychological Mechanisms Driving the Preference for Helping Identifiable Victims

Many psychological theories argue that people make judgments and decisions differently depending on how mentally and emotionally involved the decision-maker is and depending on the nature of the stimuli. Kahneman and Frederick (2002) provide an umbrella framework for these multiprocess theories, which they term "System 1" and "System 2." System 1 is the intuitive and emotional system that humans typically operate on because people rarely have time to pause and reflect on the accuracy of their gut reactions. System 2 is the slower, more deliberate system that interferes in times when people are highly motivated to and have the ability to reason through a judgment.

This general framework and more specific dual-process models are useful for understanding the identifiable victim effect. System 1 tends to dominate when the target of thought is specific and vivid (Hamilton and Sherman 1996; Sherman, Beike, and Ryalls 1999), just as people are drawn emotionally to an identified victim. They attract more attention and deeper consideration than abstract statistics, which fail to arouse an emotional response.

Moreover, such large numbers of victims can undermine the powerful emotional response to an identifiable victim. Small, Loewenstein, and Slovic (2007) found that when victim statistics (i.e., true numbers about the magnitude of various needs) were presented in charity appeals alongside an identifiable victim, donations dropped significantly and were in fact on par with appeals that only contained victim statistics. In other words, a picture and statistics are worse than just a picture.

In another study, participants were first primed to think in either an analytic or an emotional manner, and subsequently presented with an opportunity to donate. The donation appeal featured either an identifiable victim or victim statistics. In the analytic thinking conditions, the priming task consisted of solving simple word problems, while in the emotional thinking condition, the task consisted of answering questions that required participants to think with their feelings (e.g., "When you think of Princess Di, how do you feel?"). The results revealed that analytic thinking reduced average donations toward an identifiable victim—an effect similar to presenting statistics in an appeal. Yet emotional thinking failed to lift donations toward statistical victims. Such an asymmetric pattern is consistent with dual-process models of emotion and reason, which argue that emotion (part of System 1) occurs automatically, but can be overruled by deliberative reasoning (part of System 2) (Shiv and Fedorikhin 1999; Wilson and Brekke 1994; Zajonc 1980). However, it is much more difficult to get people to "feel" for statistics. These findings suggest that advocating social utility theory to policymakers and to donors—an inherently calculative approach—may lead to more economically sensible pattern of aid, but it also could dampen giving overall; without the emotional response there is little impetus to help.

One reason why people may respond to an identifiable victim in a feeling-based manner is that identification reduces psychological distance. Psychological distance refers to the connection that individuals feel to other people, places, and things. In other words, an identified victim halfway around the world may be perceived as closer and more relatable than statistical victims at the same physical distance.

In general, people tend to feel more sympathetic and more helpful toward other people who are socially closer to them—a tendency likely programmed by evolution. Kin-selection theory in biology argues that altruism depends on relatedness, or the odds that a gene in the receiver is identical by descent of a gene in the giver (Hamilton 1964). In human social reality, the exact genetic overlap between individuals is typically not observable. Therefore, humans use various heuristics to assess how "close" others are to them, such as "those in my home are kin" (Rachlin and Jones 2008; see also Railton, in this volume). It is likely that these rules, like any heuristic, get overgeneralized such that simply feeling close to someone evokes the emotional and behavioral response of a "kin" regardless of any genetic relationship.

In a compelling study, Jones and Rachlin (2006) demonstrated this subjective closeness effect by asking participants in a study to imagine a list of the one hundred people closest to them in order of closeness and to choose (hypothetically) between different allocations of money between themselves and to each of the people on the list. These lists typically started with spouses and other close relatives, followed by friends and colleagues. Results clearly showed that generosity declines with this subjective distance in a hyperbolic function.

In the Jones and Rachlin (2006) study, the list of the one hundred closest people typically begins with family, then friends, then colleagues, and acquaintances. However, people in the developed world know far more individuals than that. Therefore, the top one hundred does not include unknown others. Yet giving to charity and other prosocial action typically involves helping those with whom people have no actual relationship. Often prosocial actors do not ever learn the identities of the recipients. Yet the principles of social distance still apply. Certain anonymous victims may feel closer than others even though they may not make the top one hundred. For example, in the Milgram experiments (1974), variations of the famous experiment that involved participants believing that they were administering shocks to other participants found that when the alleged shock recipient was placed in a more (physically) distant room where they could not be heard or seen, the participant was more compliant about administering shocks than when the recipient could be seen and his or her voice heard. While other explanations could account for this result, it is consistent with the possibility that psychological distance (here triggered by physical distance) weakens caring.

To be sure, there is a great deal of evidence that factors that reduce psychological distance tend to increase caring even in anonymous interactions. For one, people care more about others when they are classified as part of the same group, even when the groups are meaningless labels (Dovidio et al. 1997). Induced similarity between beneficiary and potential helper as well as induced perspective-taking have also been shown to facilitate caring by reducing psychological distance (Stotland and Dunn 1963; Batson, Early, and Salvarani 1997). People are also more willing to help victims who suffer from the same misfortune as someone personally close to them previously suffered

(Small and Simonsohn 2008). Specifically, in experiments that manipulated "friendship" and "victimhood" and controlled for information, friendship with a victim led people to donate more to other victims of the same misfortune, but did not affect donations to victims of another, unrelated misfortune. For instance, knowing someone who suffered from cancer makes people more generous toward other cancer victims, but does not make them more generous to hurricane victims. Presumably, personal experience with a misfortune mitigates the distance from anonymous others that people typically feel and increases sympathy and caring.

In sum, there is much evidence that reducing psychological distance from anonymous victims facilitates caring. When a life becomes identified, it is more tangible and relatable. People may believe that they have true connection to the victim almost as if a real relationship exists. This feeling of psychological closeness in turn increases generosity. On the other hand, statistical lives are distant and unrelatable and thus fail to evoke a sense of connection.

Although the research on the identifiable victim effect demonstrates that people lack sympathy toward statistical victims who are socially distant and fail to evoke emotion, a recent paper demonstrates a convincing manner in which the apathy toward statistical victims can be overcome. Smith, Faro, and Burson (forthcoming) found that when a group of victims is portrayed as a coherent unit, the singularity of the unit makes the "many" appear more like "one" and thus increases caring. Specifically, when children in need were described as a family (a coherent grouping) rather than just a number of children (an incoherent grouping) they received greater donations. Similarly, when endangered animals were depicted as moving in unison or as a herd rather than a number of animals they likewise received greater donations. This further supports the special psychological power of the number one: "one child" and "one group of children" are both more effective descriptions for generating sympathy than "many children," even though a group of children is essentially equivalent to many children. This has clear implications: to raise concern for statistical lives, one must present those lives in as unified a manner as possible.

3. Are Certain Statistical Lives Valued More Than Others?

This book focuses on one specific bias that distorts sensible allocation of resources, the identifiable victim effect. As was previously mentioned, and is discussed elsewhere in this book, utilitarians would counsel that in providing aid one should donate each dollar to where it can do the most social good, irrespective of whether the beneficiary is identified or statistical. Yet behavioral evidence sometimes runs opposite to this theory—producing patterns of purportedly suboptimal giving. This chapter reviews the empirical evidence and sheds light on psychology behind the identifiable victim effect. In doing so, it helps explain why lives are valued inconsistently across victim and misfortunes. Yet it cannot explain all of the evident distortions in aid provision.

Research on the identifiable victim effect helps explain the discrepancy between giving to individuals and to large-scale disasters. However, certain large-scale disasters receive considerably more sympathy and aid than others. Specifically, devastating events, such as the 2004 Asian tsunami and the 2011 earthquake in Japan received great sums of humanitarian aid, whereas chronic states of need, such as chronic diseases and poverty, rarely witness similar outpourings of support (Epstein 2006). Indeed, private donations averaged $1,839 per person affected by Hurricane Katrina but just $10 per person affected by AIDS. In other research, I have demonstrated and discussed a different sympathy bias, which can partially account for this discrepancy termed "reference-dependent sympathy" (Small 2010). Drawing on the notion of reference dependence from judgment theories (Helson 1964; Parducci 1965), I argue that sympathy for another is a function not of the absolute state of misery, but rather from the perceived state relative to the reference point (typically the previous state). Because sympathy is based on a change, not a state, people perceived to experience loss receive greater sympathy than people with chronic misfortune.

To illustrate, consider a man who has always been homeless versus one who loses his home—both through no fault of their own. They both have an equivalent state of homelessness, but the latter has experienced a loss. According to reference-dependent sympathy, the latter tugs at our heartstrings more than the former. This provides one explanation for why sudden tragic events receive greater compassion and aid than ongoing misfortunes. It may also help explain other examples of public and government responses outside of humanitarian aid, such as the feeling of obligation to "save" people in the face of home foreclosures and layoffs and to bail out companies that have experienced large losses. In these cases, there exists a motivation to return to the reference state rather than realize the loss. Once again, the psychological tendency to restore losses may lead to inefficient resource allocation where people and firms with greater objective needs remain underfunded.

Reference-dependent sympathy provides an explanation for some otherwise peculiar real-world evidence of great sympathy for large-scale and distant disasters—that cannot be explained by the identifiable victim effect. Real-world tragic events continue to test these theories, and when they cannot, they provide ideas for new hypotheses to test.

4. Conclusion

Several lines of research in psychology reveal that people do not value lives equivalently. Research on the identifiable victim effect demonstrates that people are more sympathetic and generous toward a target that is specific and/or vivid, leading to a tendency to allocate help to a single individual rather than to large masses of victims. This tendency is contrary to the utilitarian ideal of allocating scarce resources where they can provide the greatest benefit. People often endorse social utilitarianism in the abstract or when choosing between different causes to support when the comparative impact is salient. However, in concrete situations where one cause is presented, people tend to show greater generosity when that cause tugs at their heartstrings, which is particularly common with identifiable victims.

To conclude, I hope that this chapter conveys that the identifiable victim effect is not simply one particular effect with one psychological mechanism. Rather it is a collection of related psychologies that give rise to greater attention to, and aid for, certain lives than others. That is, the evidence suggests that the extent to which a life is (a) specific, (b) vivid, and (c) represented as a high proportion of a reference group or a single unit increase generosity compared to victims who are (a) vague, (b) pallid, and (c) described as a drop in the bucket or otherwise in terms of large numbers. Each of these factors contributes to the psychological response by reducing psychological distance and by heightening the affective response. It is noteworthy that these patterns are often contradictory to the aid allocation policies that laypeople endorse in the abstract. I leave it to the health policy experts to discuss how this knowledge of human psychology can inform strategy to confront the myriad needy causes around the world that often fail to tug at the heartstrings of those with resources to share.

References

Batson, C. D., S. Early, and G. Salvarani. 1997. "Perspective Taking: Imagining How Another Feels versus Imagining How You Would Feel." *Personality and Social Psychology Bulletin* 23 (7): 751–58.

Bentham, J. [1843] 1948. *An Introduction to the Principles of Morals and Legislation.* Oxford: Basil Blackwell.

Dovidio, J. F., S. K. Gaertner, A. Validzic, K. Matoka, B. Johnson, and S. Frazier. 1997. "Extending the Benefits of Recategorization: Evaluations, Self-Disclosure, and Helping." *Journal of Experimental Social Psychology* 33 (4): 401–20.

Epstein, K. 2006. "Crisis Mentality: Why Sudden Emergencies Attract More Funds Than Do Chronic Conditions, and How Nonprofits Can Change That." *Stanford Social Innovation Review,* 4 (1), 46–55.

Featherstonhaugh, D., P. Slovic, S. M. Johnson, and J. Friedrich. 1997. "Insensitivity to the Value of Human Life: A Study of Psychophysical Numbing." *Journal of Risk and Uncertainty* 14: 283–300.

Galak, J., D. A. Small, and A. Stephen. 2011. "Microfinance Decision Making: A Field Study of Prosocial Lending." *Journal of Marketing Research* 48: 130–37.

Hamilton, D. L., and S. J. Sherman. 1996. "Perceiving Persons and Groups." *Psychol. Rev.* 103 (2): 336–55.

Hamilton, W. D. 1964. "The Genetical Evolution of Social Behavior." *Journal of Theoretical Biology* 7: 1-52.
Helson, H. 1964. *Adaptation-Level Theory*. New York: Harper and Row.
Hsee, C. K., and Y. Rottenstreich. 2004. "Music, Pandas, and Muggers: On the Affective Psychology of Value." *Journal of Experimental Psychology: General* 133 (1): 25-30.
Jenni, K. E., and G. F. Loewenstein. 1997. "Explaining the 'Identifiable Victim Effect.'" *Journal of Risk and Uncertainty* 14: 235-57.
Jones, B., and H. Rachlin. 2006. "Social Discounting." *Psychological Science* 17: 283-86.
Kahneman, D., and S. Frederick. 2002. "Representativeness Revisited: Attribute Substitution in Intuitive Judgment." In *Heuristics and Biases*, edited by Thomas Gilovich, Dale Griffin, and Daniel Kahneman, 49-81. New York: Cambridge University Press.
Kogut, T., and I. Ritov. 2005a. "The 'Identified Victim' Effect: An Identified Group or Just an Individual?" *Journal of Behavioral Decision Making* 18 (3): 157-67.
———. 2005b. "The Singularity Effect of Identified Victims in Separate and Joint Evaluation." *Organizational Behavior and Human Decision Processes* 97 (2): 106-16.
Loewenstein, G., and D. A. Small. 2007. "The Scarecrow and the Tinman: The Vicissitudes of Human Sympathy and Caring." *Review of General Psychology* 11 (2): 112-26.
Milgram, S. 1974. *Obedience to Authority: An Experimental View*. New York: Harper and Row.
Mill, J. S. [1863] 1906. *Utilitarianism*. Chicago: University of Chicago Press.
Parducci, A. 1965. "Category Judgment: A Range-Frequency Model." *Psychological Review* 72 (6): 407-18.
Rachlin, H., and B. A. Jones. 2008. "Altruism among Relatives and Non-relatives." *Behavioral Processes* 79: 120-23.
Schelling, T. C. 1968. "The Life You Save May Be Your Own." In *Problems in Public Expenditure Analysis*, edited by S. B. Chase, 127-62. Washington, DC: Brookings Institute.
Sherman, S. J., D. R. Beike, and K. R. Ryalls. 1999. "Dual-Processing Accounts of Inconsistencies in Responses to General versus Specific Cases." In *Dual-Process Theories in Social Psychology*, edited by S. Chaiken and Y. Trope, 203-27. New York: Guilford Press.
Shiv, B., and A. Fedorikhin. 1999. "Heart and Mind in Conflict: The Interplay of Affect and Cognition in Consumer Decision Making." *Journal of Consumer Research* 26: 278-92.
Small, D. A. 2010. "Reference-Dependent Sympathy." *Organizational Behavior and Human Decision Processes* 112 (2): 151-60.
Small, D. A., and G. Loewenstein. 2003. "Helping a Victim or Helping the Victim: Altruism and Identifiability." *Journal of Risk and Uncertainty* 26 (1): 5-16.
Small, D. A., and U. Simonsohn. 2008. "Friends of Victims: The Impact of Personal Relationships with Victims on Generosity toward Others." *Journal of Consumer Research* 35: 532-42.
Small, D. A., G. Loewenstein, and P. Slovic. 2007. "Sympathy and Callousness: The Impact of Deliberative Thought on Donations to Identifiable and Statistical Victims." *Organizational Behavior and Human Decision Processes* 102 (2): 143-53.
Smith, R. W., D. Faro, and K. A. Burson. 2013. "More for the Many: The Influence of Entitativity on Charitable Giving." *Journal of Consumer Research* 39 (5), 961-76.
Stiglitz, J. E. 1990. "Peer Monitoring and Credit Markets." *World Bank Economics Review* 4 (3): 351-66.
Stotland, E., and R. E. Dunn. 1963. "Empathy, Self-Esteem, and Birth Order." *Journal of Abnormal and Social Psychology* 66 (6): 532-40.

Varian, H. R. 1990. "Monitoring Agents with Other Agents." *Journal of Institutional and Theoretical Economics* 146: 153–74.

Wilson, T. D., and N. C. Brekke. 1994. "Mental Contamination and Mental Correction: Unwanted Influences on Judgments and Evaluations." *Psychological Bulletin* 116: 117–42.

Yunus, M. 1999. *Banker to the Poor*. New York: Public Affairs.

Zajonc, R. 1980. "Feeling and Thinking: Preferences Need No Inferences." *American Psychologist* 35: 151–75.

2 }

"Dual-Process" Models of the Mind and the "Indentifiable Victim Effect"

Peter Railton

1. Introduction: An Asymmetry

The question of "statistical victims" could not be more central to debates over the ethics and politics of healthcare. An extensive body of evidence suggests that people generally take more seriously the plight of actual, identifiable individual victims of harm than that of unidentified, indeterminate, or merely possible victims—so-called "statistical victims." For example, college students who had just received five one-dollar bills in payment for filling out questionnaires as part of a psychology experiment were asked if they wished to return some of this money to make a donation to Habitat for Humanity. Those who were told the donations would help provide housing for a family that *has been selected* gave more of their five dollars than those who were told that a family *will be selected* (Small and Lowenstein 2003). This "identifiable victim effect" is well known to charities, journalists, and politicians. Vividly presenting the situation of an actual individual can evoke a stronger response than abstract statistics, even when the statistics attest to the fate of a greater number.

This effect appears to be especially prominent in "intuitive" decision-making—decisions that are made more or less spontaneously, without explicit consultation of rules or principles. Neither is this the only apparent rational deficiency of intuitive decision-making—many others have been identified (see, for example, Kahneman and Tversky 2000). Since "intuitions" nonetheless seem inevitably to come into play when we deliberate about matters of policy, it behooves us to inquire into their possible origin and nature. We must ask whether, once we have a better understanding how they arise or what they might reflect, we have reason to place less confidence in them.

Certainly the "statistical" or "identifiable victim effect" appears to be ripe for such interrogation.[1] It seems obvious that the harms borne by future victims or victims whose identity happens to be unknown to us are not for that reason alone any less severe; neither is our ability to ameliorate their condition for that reason alone any less real and important. This should be especially worrisome in matters of individual medical care and general health policy, since it is impossible to discuss such matters sensibly without facing trade-offs between actual, identifiable harms and benefits, on the one hand, and harms and benefits that are (as yet) unknown or "merely" potential, on the other. Of course, to explain the origin of intuitive assessments is a *descriptive* project, within the domain of the social sciences, whereas inquiring into their credibility is a *normative* enterprise, more properly in the domain of epistemology or ethics. It is, however, part of epistemic or ethical inquiry to look into the presuppositions or processes underlying how we think and feel. So it is in that spirit that I—no expert in psychology, sociology, economics, or health science—will be scrutinizing what appears to be the predominant form of explanation currently on offer of the "identifiable victim effect," and suggesting an alternative. My conclusions should therefore be seen as conditional: if the empirical claims upon which I am basing my arguments are right (or near enough so), then we have reason to make certain normative inferences. While I will, of course, be making my best effort to be responsive to the empirical evidence of which I am aware, there is so much of which I am unaware that my prescriptions should be taken *cum granis salis*.

2. Explaining the "Identifiable Victim Effect": Dual-Process Models of the Mind

Recently, interest has grown in giving an explanation of the "identifiable victim effect" as an affective rather than purely cognitive phenomenon. Descriptions of identifiable individual victims are thought to arouse different affective responses from accounts of merely possible, abstractly described, unidentified, or indeterminate victims. One very plausible thought here is that it is easier to empathize with a victim the more vividly one can imagine her plight. However, the bare information that a beneficiary has been selected versus will

---

[1] In reality, there might be a number of "effects" at work—actual vs. possible harm, vividness vs. abstractness, identifiability vs. anonymity of the victim(s), absolute vs. relative numbers, probabilities vs. other magnitudes, and so on. For simplicity, I will usually speak in what follows of the "identifiable victim effect," though occasionally these various "effects" will need to be distinguished. For reasons that will emerge below, "identified victim effect" seems to me a more apt generic expression. I will follow the (I'm afraid) annoying practice of writing "identifiable" or "statistical victim effect" in scare quotes, since it seems to me we should, for present purposes, hold open the question of how appropriate these labels are.

be selected—which Small and Lowenstein (2003) found to elicit an "identifiable victim effect"—does not seem to invite much greater vividness of imagining. As daydreamers and planners alike know, mere futurity is not a barrier to imagination—indeed, recent work suggests that mental simulation of future possibilities is a core function of the brain (Buckner and Carroll 2007; Seligman et al. 2013).

More direct evidence comes from experimental studies. One study found no evidence that empathy is playing an important role in the effect (Kogut and Ritov 2007), while another found no significant correlation between felt distress or sympathy and the magnitude of the effect (Friedrich and McGuire 2010). A different set of experiments found a correlation between willingness to contribute, on the one hand, and distress and sympathy expressed after the fact, on the other (Small, Lowenstein, and Slovic 2007). But a more controlled replication of these experiments suggests that the variation is mediated by differences in cognitive styles between the more intuitive and more calculative (Friedrich and McGuire 2010).

This last result suggests a different way in which affect might play a role in the effect—it could be that affective responses are different in kind from more cognitive responses. In particular, affect might be moved by identifying information in ways that displace rational calculation. An explanation of this kind promises to explain a number of curious features of the effect. For example, Kogut and Ritov (2004) found that a group of experimental subjects asked to make a donation that would benefit an identified single victim on average gave larger amounts than a similar group asked to make a donation to benefit an identified group of victims. Even when subjects were offered both options in a nonexclusive choice, their average contribution was no larger for the group than for the individual. Only when both options were offered in a forced choice did subjects' average contribution to the group exceed that for a single individual victim. Since affective states are viewed as qualitative, "holistic," or "blunt" in character, insensitivity to the numbers involved might be expected to result. Only when subjects are explicitly required to contemplate a choice between aiding an individual and aiding a group does quantitative, analytic, or expected-value-based thought come into play, bringing the difference in number to the fore, mitigating the affective effect. Kogut and Ritov (2004) conclude:

> The lack of sufficient sensitivity to quantity stems, most likely, from a decision process reflecting primarily the respondents' attitude, or emotional reaction toward the target, rather than a rational, quantitative calculation of the intervention's utility. (citing Kahneman, Ritov, and Schkade 1999, 106)

Small, Lowenstein, and Slovic (2007) offer a similar diagnosis in similar cases, invoking the idea of an "affect heuristic" in which individuals implicitly rely upon their affective reactions to simulated outcomes rather than calculation of expected value:

> when making a decision to donate money to a cause, most people do not calculate the expected benefit of their donation. Rather, choices are made intuitively, based upon spontaneous affective reactions. (Slovic et al. 2002, 144; see Schwartz and Clore 1983)

Such affect-based explanations of the identifiable victim effect have recently come to be seen as instances of a more general "dual-process" approach to the organization of the mind. Hsee and Rottenstreich (2004) write:

> Recent literature identifies two distinct modes of thought, one deliberate and rule-based, the other associative and affect based (e.g., Chaiken and Trope, 1999; Epstein, 1994; Kahneman and Frederick, 2002; Sloman, 1996). Building on such dual-process models, we distinguish between two psychological processes by which people might assess the value of a particular target: valuation by calculation and valuation by feeling. . . . Specifically, we suggest that under valuation by calculation, changes in scope [e.g., number, magnitude, probability] have relatively constant influence throughout the entire range. . . . However, we suggest that under valuation by feeling, value is highly sensitive to the absence or presence of a stimulus (e.g., a change from 0 to some scope) but is largely insensitive to further variations in scope. (23)

Here, for example, is how Small, Lowenstein, and Slovic (2006) use the dual-process model to get more theoretical purchase on the mental processes underlying identifiable victim effect:

> Recent dual process models in social cognition identify two distinct modes of thought: one deliberate and calculative and the other affective. . . . The identifiable victim effect, it seems, may result from divergent modes of thought, with greater felt sympathy for identifiable victims because they invoke the affective system. (144)

In dual-process models the two "modes" of thought normally operate in parallel in the mind, though they can yield conflicting results for a given stimulus. The spontaneous, largely implicit, affect-based "System 1" is seen as "ancient" (that is, shared with our proximate mammalian ancestors), "automatic," and "very fast" (Haidt 2007). Moreover, according to the thesis of "affective primacy" (Zajonc 1980, 1984), the affective mode of mental processing comes online very early in the perceptual stream, coding incoming information with positive or negative emotional valence and influencing our interpretation of the stimulus before conscious, declarative thought comes into play. As a result, System 1 can yield "instinctual" or "automatic" responses, "gut feelings," that are insensitive to variations in the benefits or harms that a more deliberative, analytic mode of thought would detect. Jonathan Haidt, for example, argues that subjects reading a scenario involving sibling incest experience a "flash of disgust" that leads them to condemn the action morally, ignoring the fact that the incident as described was consensual and led to no real harm (Haidt 2001, 2007). The "deliberate and calculative" "System 2," by contrast, is "phylogenetically newer, slower, and motivationally weaker." It can succeed in critiquing or overriding prompt or "automatic" emotional assessments—that is, reflective "evaluation by calculation" can trump spontaneous "evaluation by feeling." But since most choice is spontaneous rather than deliberative, this sort of rational correction is the exception rather than the rule. And often, when System 2 does get involved in choice, it comes online after the fact, elaborating post hoc rationalizations of our spontaneous responses or actions, rather than supplying independent guidance (Haidt 2001, 2007). Daniel Kahneman's recent book, *Thinking, Fast and Slow* (2011), deploys a dual-process model to explain a very wide range of otherwise puzzling thought or behavior. In his view, the fast System 1 includes "innate skills that we share with other animals," but "has little understanding of logic and statistics" (21, 24), and this accounts for the persistent failure of experimental subjects to deliver rational responses when presented with a number of tasks involving probability or expected value. The slow, effortful, deliberative, rule-based System 2 typically comes into play only when there is greater felt need for cognition, for example, when "intuitive" responses conflict or fail in practical terms.

A prediction of the dual-process account is that, when more reflective modes of thought are primed in an experimental setting, this should encourage more quantitative, rule-based responses and diminish the "identifiable victim effect," whereas when emotion is primed, the effect should increase. And this is indeed what has been observed (Hsee and Rottenstreich 2004; Kogut and Ritov 2004; Small and Lowenstein 2003).

In sum, on dual-process accounts of the mind, our spontaneous evaluative "intuitions" are far from being what moral philosophers might have supposed. They are manifestations of "blunt" or "push-button" emotional responses (Greene 2013), not manifestations of an underlying, principled moral sense or rational competency.

2.1. STATISTICAL ANIMALS

The dual-process model of the mind has won increasingly wide acceptance in psychology and neuroscience, and its use to explain the identifiable victim effect appears to be empirically and theoretically well motivated. Moreover, this explanation would be highly relevant to our question about the normative assessment of the "intuitions" found in the "identifiable victim effect": "automatic," "push-button" emotional responses that "have little understanding of logic and statistics" and tend to preempt or crowd out more rational thought are hardly the sorts of responses to defer to when deliberating about complex questions of resource allocation or healthcare policy.

So let us examine the dual-process model and what bearing it might have on the explanation of "intuitive" assessment a bit more carefully. For this purpose, an ecological perspective might be a good starting point. If System 1 has its origin in our animal ancestry, what sorts of problems did our animal ancestors have to solve, and what capacities might therefore have been evolved in order to solve them?

Animals live on the margins of existence. Thanks to competition, they face recurring scarcity of nutrients, warmth, water, protection from predation, and access to mates or cooperation partners. Animals who solve these problems stand a much better chance of prospering and leaving progeny than those who do not. Efficiency and effectiveness are therefore at a premium, and any bit of behavior, from the simple movement of an eye tracking a moving object to picking a fight in order to win a mating partner, is likely to be more efficient and effective if it is based upon a more accurate anticipation of what will happen next. Hence, there has been relentless selection for abilities to form and be guided by accurate expectations of the physical and social environment and its possibilities and perils—at least within a time horizon in which animals can achieve better-than-chance prediction (on animal time horizons, see Suddendorf and Corballis 2010). Since an animal's physical and social environment tends to undergo continuing change, no fixed set of expectations will suffice—updating expectations and adjusting behavior to take advantage of fresh opportunities or avoid newly emerging risks is a core task of any intelligent animal making its way in the world. Predators and prey, for example, are locked in an arms race in which the least anticipatory cues of the other's next movement—such as variations of a few degrees in the other's head position—can be seized upon and used to promote successful predation or evasion.

Perhaps it seems preposterous to imagine animals as guided by brains designed to make efficient use of information to form forward expectations of possible risks and benefits. Aren't animals "stimulus bound" creatures of instinct, association, and "automatic" habit—incapable of dissociating themselves from the present to anticipate conditions that do not yet exist?

It appears not. Consider the behavior of food-caching birds and mammals. Northern food-caching birds face a real risk of freezing overnight and would have disappeared long ago if they were not able to forgo consuming food on the spot even when hungry in order to cache food for retrieval near sunset. While there is an "innate disposition" to cache food, the deployment of this capacity must be responsive to continuing variation in nutritional needs, the qualities and quantities of the food available, and the risk or effort involved in obtaining them. For example, western scrub-jays keep track of where they have cached perishable worms versus imperishable nuts, and of how long the worms have been cached, retrieving them before they spoil. If prevented from foraging for several days, long enough for the worms to spoil, the jays will shift their retrieving behavior to favor nuts. If this pattern continues, they learn not to cache worms at all, but to eat them on the spot while continuing to cache nuts (for a summary of results, see Raby and Clayton 2009).

Or consider neurological observations of a rat foraging in the classic T-maze beloved by behaviorists. Microelectrode recording of neuron firing rates and patterns in the hippocampus and cortex suggest that the rat has "grid" and "place" neurons that build up a persisting spatial representation of the maze over the course of the rat's explorations and trial runs. This multidimensional representation has substantial autonomy from local stimulation. For example, during REM sleep after a day of training and during awake resting periods, this representation can be observed to be repeatedly activated. Activation can spread forward or backward, and there is often greater activation in areas where the animal has spent less time—patterns of mental simulation opposite what one would predict for associative learners or creatures of habit, but just what one would expect in efficient statistical learners modeling the maze (Foster and Wilson 2006; Ji and Wilson 2007). As a result of this overnight or resting activity, rats can learn without novel external stimulus or reinforcement, showing improvement in speed and effectiveness of performance in the maze. Intriguingly, when the rat is back in the maze and has reached a choice point, activation in its spatial representation can be observed to spread ahead of its current location, sweeping out the alternate paths with an intensity of neuron firing that reflects previously learned probabilities and magnitudes of reward and predicts actual choice of path (Johnson and Redish 2007).

Further insight into animal modeling of the environment comes from microelectrode studies of reinforcement learning in macaques, which indicate separate neural encoding of information about the probability versus the magnitude of rewards, with fine-grained quantitative variation in firing rates that increases across the interval from probability zero to probability one (Schultz 2002; Tobler et al. 2006). Affective responses thus show calibrated "attunement" and "reattunement" to a changing environment. For example, responses to negative stimuli in rats are not a simple matter of "button pushing," but rather are registered on an "affective keyboard"; the proportion "tuned" to negative versus positive events varies in response to variations in levels of risk in the environment (Reynolds and Berridge 2008).

Animal learning thus turns out not to be the associative entrenchment of stimulus-triggered motor habits, but a flexible, quantitatively precise process by which animals selectively attend to and utilize information from experience to develop expectation-based models of their environment and its prospects and perils relative to meeting their physical and social needs. This picture of animal learning helps explain an ecological phenomenon long observed across a wide range of species: in natural settings and laboratories alike, animals can relatively quickly develop nearly optimal foraging patterns, balancing nutrition requirements, energy costs, risks, the need to explore for new sources, and so on (Dugatkin

2004). Near-optimality in behavior has also been observed in the selection of prey, mates, and cooperation partners (Krebs et al. 1977; Melis, Hare, and Tomasello 2006). Balancing the many variables in play in such complex activities is an enormously complicated computational problem, yet millions of generations of natural selection appear to have designed animal learning systems to solve such problems efficiently and effectively, managing a good approximation of Bayesian learning and decision-making (Courville, Daw, and Touretzky 2005). The affect and reward system we inherit from the animals, then, is hardly stimulus-bound, statistically naive, or insensitive to variations in quantity—quite the opposite.

2.2. SYSTEM 1 AND SYSTEM 2 REDUX

Brain-imaging studies of humans suggest that our inherited, enlarged, and better-connected affect and reward system plays a similar role in encoding information about probability and value—for example, as observed in gambling experiments and in choice behavior in foraging tasks (Kolling et al. 2012; Preuschoff, Bossaerts, and Quartz 2006). Moreover, like the rats, we humans appear to engage in spontaneous offline simulation of possibilities when resting or sleeping (Taylor et al. 1998; Buckner and Carroll 2007; Mason et al. 2007).

The "skills . . . we share with animals" would thus appear to include flexible, sophisticated, quantitatively accurate capacities for forming prospective representations or *forward models* of the possible costs and benefits of potential acts and outcomes. These expectation-based models are continuously updated through discrepancy-reduction learning, and they serve to guide behavior intelligently even in the absence of conscious deliberation and planning. Truly exceptional athletes, for example, appear to differ from very good athletes less in their motor competencies, than in the richness, speed, and accuracy of their forward models of competitive situations (Yarrow, Brown, and Krakauer 2009).

Why, then, are we so bad at probabilistic estimation and calculation, as Kahneman and Amos Tversky, and many in their wake, have repeatedly shown (Kahneman and Tversky 1979, 2000; Kahneman 2003)? Since the forward models spontaneously constructed and updated by our affect and reward system are largely implicit, we have no direct access to them. The statistical competency they embody, therefore, is not available on command. Experimental subjects, for example, appear to be particularly poor at estimating conditional probabilities. But even 8-month-old babies, as yet unable to speak and years before they can carry out controlled, deliberative reasoning, can discriminate probable from improbable sequences of sounds in English, in effect implicitly computing accurate conditional probabilities on the basis of experienced relative frequencies (Aslin, Saffran, and Newport 1998). Moreover, they pay greater attention to the improbable sequences—again, the sign of effective statistical learning rather than associative entrenchment of habits (Saffran, Aslin, and Newport, 1996). The rules or norms figuring in language and communication are intricate and context-dependent. Yet virtually every child growing up in a society will acquire a rather high degree of linguistic and communicative competence, supporting fluent, spontaneous speech and shared "linguistic intuitions." So, to a greater or lesser degree, will a plumber, farmer, physical therapist, or chess player acquire the complex implicit knowledge structures needed to practice these skills with a reasonable level of fluency and success. To the conscious mind, the exercise of these acquired skills and competencies is "intuitive" and qualitative—a given move in a competitive game, a particular response to an awkward social situation, or a particular spoken sentence will "feel right" or "feel wrong" depending upon its fit with the patterns and expectations embedded in our implicit models. This will be experienced as a "noncalculative" or "nonrational" response, even though it might be the product of highly calculative, reasons-sensitive processes.

By contrast, System 2 carries out explicit, effortful deliberation or calculation. For this reason, it operates under rather severe limits of attention, concentration, control, sequencing, and computation. Ask us explicitly to estimate or calculate or utilize a probability in an experiment based upon word problems, and we typically will have no choice but to rely upon this system. As a result, we tend to rely upon "heuristics" or "rules of thumb" to attempt to simplify the estimation or calculation, but these will make us liable to systematic errors. For example, in "probability matching," human subjects given a set of examples or choices in which the frequency of *F*s versus *G*s, or of winning with choice *A* versus *B*, is 80% versus 20% are asked to predict how one should classify a set of new examples or make the next choices; they tend to say that one should divide the sample or choices 80:20. This is a nonoptimal response—proper Bayesian reasoning would have them favor categorizing as *F* or choosing *A* in each new case. Unlike humans, animals tend to solve this problem correctly. Does this show an implicit system bad at statistics, or an explicit system working with a heuristic? When Shanks and colleagues (2002) allowed implicit human statistical learning to have a chance by doing multiple runs of such problems with meaningful feedback (2002), they found that humans, too, shifted away from probability matching. Similar results have been obtained with statistical learning and the famous "Monty Hall problem" (Friedman 1998). It appears that when System 1 can be brought into play experientially through prompt and accurate feedback, some of the probabilistic fallacies generated by explicit thought in System 2 can be counteracted by acting "intuitively." Meteorologists, regulars at the horse-track, and top-flight bridge players have ample feedback and high motivation to estimate probabilities accurately, and they show very good calibration of expectations. Those in professions such as emergency medicine, where feedback is typically belated and incomplete, show much poorer calibration (for a summary, see Liley and Rakow 2010).

The special strength of System 2 might not be the ability to calculate statistics or expected value—System 1 appears very capable of handling such tasks implicitly, whereas people's explicit efforts to assign probabilities have well-known liabilities. Rather, where System 2 has a comparative advantage is in overcoming two crucial limitations of purely statistical learning. First, statistical learning does not have an inherent mechanism for the formulation or testing of novel concepts, hypotheses, or methods. Yet if humans are distinctive for anything within the animal world, it is for their ability to innovate in these ways. It is chiefly by such cultural innovation that humans have—for better or worse—distanced themselves so far from their highly intelligent primate relatives, who face extinction owing to loss of their habitat while we have no fixed habitat. The conscious, conceptual apparatus in which to pose—much less solve—the questions of social choice that face us in health policy is not to be found among the great apes. In contrast to the largely implicit and inarticulate knowledge contained within System 1, the conscious, language-based character of typical System 2 thought makes it possible for individuals to share experience and learn by explicit instruction, greatly accelerating learning and expanding the "time depth" of knowledge. Second, the controlled character of reasoning in System 2 makes it possible to build from "intuitive" starting points much more elaborate models of ourselves and our world, greatly enlarging the "time horizon" of planning and choice. Our implicit System 1 can count and calculate, keep track of physiological variables and social interactions, and form complex forward models that guide decision and action, closely approximating the prescriptions of Bayesian epistemology and decision theory. But System 1 would never by itself yield Bayesian epistemology and decision theory, or, for that matter, the idea of actuarially sound social insurance, global climate change, or democratic political institutions. System 1 can make us efficient, effective, sensible, and sociable hominids, but it took the yoking together of System 1 and System 2 to transform such hominids into the creatures we now know as modern humans.

3. Implicit Social Competence and the "Identifiable" or "Statistical Victim Effect"

Understanding the differences in attitude toward identified versus unidentified or merely possible victims in terms of a conflict between Reason (System 2) and Passion (System 1) is an attractive idea, but it runs afoul of our emerging understanding of the nature and function of the affective system. Once we come to see System 1 (the affective system) as designed for experience-based construction of expectation-based evaluative models of situations, actions, and outcomes, we will no longer see the same tension between passionate "valuation by feeling" and rational "valuation by calculation." Instead, System 1 emerges as a core part of our capacity for apt responsiveness to reasons. But where, then, does this leave the "statistical" or "identifiable victim effect"? The effect does not seem entirely attributable to fallacies of self-conscious deliberation—as we noted above, if one primes more deliberative modes of thought, the effect can be reduced or eliminated, whereas priming more affective modes of thought enhances it. How, then, does this square with the account just given of System 1 as generating experience-attuned expected values? Might the effect actually reflect a well-attuned assessment of expected value after all? How could that be, if the amount of need and the amount of aid would be the same whether the victim is actual or future, or identified versus unidentified? Let's identify two dimensions of the expected-value problem that confronts "intuition" in the case of identified versus unidentified victims: estimation of the probability of benefit or harm and estimation of its magnitude.

3.1. "INTUITIVE" ESTIMATION OF THE PROBABILITY OF BENEFIT OR HARM

An ecologically valid, statistically savvy forward model of social situations will, of course, reckon subjective or epistemic probability in its assessments. At first, it might seem that the epistemic probabilities must be equal in identified versus unidentified, or actual versus possible cases. After all, the scenarios given to experimental subjects typically do not stipulate the existence of any uncertainty. Yet in the actual world, the absence of identifying information, or the fact that an outcome is possible rather than actual (so that certain steps in the process of bringing it about remain to be completed), is reliably related to lesser certainty about the putative benefit or harm. The implicit model, then, would use the existence of identifying information or actual victims to estimate a higher probability of the harm (or benefit of helping), and thus would, other things equal, underwrite a stronger disposition to contribute or "willingness to pay."

Our implicit system of expectation formation tends to seize upon whatever shreds of evidence might have some predictive value. (This has been demonstrated in the animal literature, in which animals in reinforcement learning cue their behavior to the most predictive cues [Rescorla 1988].) Consider in this light the results reported by Small and Lowenstein (2003), discussed at the outset. In this experiment, subjects are told either that a family in need *has been selected* or that it *will be selected* to receive a benefit toward which one is invited to contribute—in this case, a house built by Habitat for Humanity. How might this tiny difference in wording make any difference to a socially competent person's willingness to make a contribution? In ordinary life, we cannot count on things happening according to plan, and there is therefore an informational asymmetry between hearing that a family has been versus will be identified to receive a benefit. One has only to ask about the difference between hearing that one's promotion has just been approved by the college versus will soon be approved. *Will soon be* remains, in the real world, contingent in a way *has just been* is not—something can still happen. That is why junior faculty are on tenterhooks until they hear that the college has approved their promotion—even when they have been assured by knowledgeable colleagues that their case will undoubtedly go through. Or consider the difference between being told by a neighbor that "some people" agree with him that you should mow your lawn more often, as opposed to being given the identities of these individuals—which has higher credibility? An evolutionary theorist would add what we already implicitly know as social beings: asking for help in one's own name is a riskier strategy than asking anonymously, since it renders one publicly vulnerable, thereby sending a more expensive—hence more credible—signal of need. Since the expected value of a contribution is a function of the probability of a benefit (or harm) as well as its magnitude, an ecologically valid, statistically savvy forward model would, other things equal, generate a higher expected value for contributing to help (or prevent harm to) an identified victim.

3.2. INTUITIVE ESTIMATION OF THE MAGNITUDE OF BENEFIT OR HARM

How would an ecologically valid, statistically savvy forward model estimate the magnitude of a benefit or harm based upon whether the victim is or is not identified? Just as we implicitly know that making an identifiable request for help is a riskier signal than seeking help anonymously, we know that it is more of a harm to the individual in need when his personal request for help is spurned. The misfortune of failing to receive needed assistance is augmented by a loss of face and social signal of rejection. It might "look bad" for the members of a community when an anonymous request for help is rejected, but this is a diffuse effect. By contrast, it unquestionably "looks bad" for an individual when his identifiable personal appeal for help goes unanswered. Moreover, the harm done by refusal would also be more salient and intense for an identifiable individual making a request on his own behalf, as opposed to making a request on behalf of an identifiable group to which he belongs. Someone with tacit competence in social modeling and valuation would thus feel greater "intuitive" pressure to give assistance to an identified victim. Indeed, as we noted above, Kogut and Ritov (2007) found that, when the cases were presented separately, identifiable individuals received greater contributions than identifiable groups.

Of course, these interactive social considerations might seem irrelevant given that the stipulations in the examples posed to experimental subjects typically include little or no social context. But the way an individual views a request is not exhausted by what is stipulated—in making an "intuitive" choice, the tacit social competence an experimental subject brings to the choice task will tend to seize upon small clues in the information given, and combine them with much wider implicit social knowledge to fill out and evaluate the simulated alternatives.

At the conscious level this sort of "intuitive" simulation and evaluation will rarely be experienced as an expected-value calculation. As Kahneman, Ritov, and Schkade (1999) write, "when making a decision to donate money to a cause, most people do not calculate the expected benefit of their donation. Rather, choices are made intuitively, based upon spontaneous affective reactions" (144). Such spontaneous affective reactions might be no more articulate than a stronger positive feeling toward giving aid in one kind of case as opposed to another, or a stronger negative feeling toward failing to give. Such a summative positive or negative "intuitive sense," of greater or lesser strength, perhaps colored by one or another emotion, is typical of the way that implicit simulation and evaluation manifest themselves in consciousness. Over the course of experience, we acquire a "feel" for the things we know, and an increasingly sensitive and effective "feel" for that which we know well. It is possible to call this sort of reliance upon "valuation by feeling" the "affect heuristic" or "simulation heuristic" at work (Kahneman and Tversky 1982; Slovic et al. 2002). But on the account of the affective system given here, "valuation by feeling" is not to be contrasted with "valuation by calculation" (cf. Hsee and Rottenstreich 2004)—rather, the complex array of "intuitions" and "feelings" we use to navigate the social world are typically conscious expressions of tacit "valuation by calculation."

3.3. LOOKING FORWARD

Should we therefore simply accept the "intuitive" judgments displaying "identifiable" or "statistical victim effect"? No, but we might want to listen more carefully to them once we have a better idea of what they might convey by way of tacit social knowledge.

Any individual's "intuitions" will reflect his limited and often unrepresentative experience, his partiality and personal aims, his capacity to project himself imaginatively into novel situations or other's shoes, his inventiveness, and the depth of his understanding. Conscious, controlled thought has distinctive contributions to make in contending with these limitations, as do social processes of sharing information, expertise, norms, and deliberation. "Intuition" needs the discipline of controlled thought to mitigate overgeneralization from one's own experience or excessive confidence in one's ability to understand what life is like for others, or will be like in the future. The large questions we face when thinking of how best to meet people's needs for assistance or healthcare will require heavy reliance on these more disciplined ways of thinking. This does not, however, move us beyond "intuition," for conscious decision-making relies in countless ways upon an "intuitive" sense of things.

Do we therefore end up in the same place as the more orthodox accounts of the "identifiable victim effect" with which we began? Not really. The difference can perhaps most readily be seen in the picture that emerges of how to go forward in practice. If affective responses are responsive to evidence and reflect underlying social competencies, rather than "push-button" responses driven by "heuristics," then the way is open to improve their evidence and increase their competence. People, we know, can acquire greater competency in a given domain when they gain more extensive and variegated experience, can make use of what they learn, and benefit from clear feedback. That is the moral of skill-learning generally, from language acquisition to playing championship bridge. Research on implicit stereotyping, for example, suggests that an effective way of reducing one's stereotypes is to have actual experiences of working toward shared goals with individuals in the stigmatized group (Blincoe and Harris 2009). But how to give people the relevant kinds of experience in the domain of something like healthcare policy?

We should take a page from the book of those most dedicated to the development of skills and accurate and effective forward models. Plane crashes and near-crashes are, thankfully, rare, so flight trainers do not simply wait for pilots to have such experiences in order to develop the relevant skills. We create simulators where they can practice intensively, to undergo the experiences necessary to have the right intuitive responses when emergencies do arise. Presidential elections are also rare, thankfully, so President Obama's campaign staff did not wait until November to see how things might turn out. Instead they developed an elaborate method of running countless simulations of the election throughout the campaign, using as much grassroots statistical data as they could gather, and updating daily. As a result, they got a clearer and more accurate picture of what would happen on Election Day in time to do something about it in advance.

The same ingenuity can be applied to improve decision-making in health policy. We will get clearer and more accurate thinking, and more sensible decisions, when we find ways of providing voters and decision-makers experience with actual or simulated healthcare choices and outcomes in terms accessible to System 1 as well as System 2. Since System 1 is evolved to take as input situational experience and episodic memory, this means that "choice simulators," like flight simulators, must provide concrete representations that mimic real choice situations and provide the feedback of mimicking real outcomes from choices made.

The daily life of health professionals delivers them experience with some fraction of the healthcare world, but not all. Specialist doctors working in private clinics do not have the daily experience of nurses or psychiatric social workers in inner-city public hospitals, and vice versa. Physicians do not have the experience of actuaries, and vice versa. And when we turn to the wider electorate, the experiential base in healthcare policy is yet more limited. People's formidable learning capacities in the social domain call for respect. People learn new languages, new cultures, and new social skills day in and day out. In the animal world, this is unprecedented. We can learn to work with, rather than against, this human capacity to learn. But it will not happen if we continue to think that normative intuitions arising from the affective system "know little of statistics or logic" or are "insensitive to quantity."

Acknowledgments

I would like to thank my coparticipants in the workshop on the "identifiable victim effect" at the Harvard School of Public Health, the editors of this volume, and anonymous referees for very helpful comments.

References

Aslin, R. N., J. R. Saffran, and E. L. Newport. 1998. "Computation of Conditional Probability Statistics by 8-Month-Old Infants." *Psychological Science* 9: 321–24.

Blincoe, S., and M. J. Harris. 2009. "Prejudice Reduction in White Students: Comparing Three Conceptual Approaches." *Journal of Diversity in Higher Education* 2: 232–42.

Buckner, R., and D. Carroll. 2007. "Self-Projection and the Brain." *Trends in Cognitive Sciences* 11: 49–57.

Chaiken, S., and Y. Trope, eds. 1999. *Dual-Process Theories in Social Psychology.* New York: Guilford Press.

Courville, A. C., N. D. Daw, and D. S. Touretzky. 2006. "Bayesian Theories of Conditioning in a Changing World." *Trends in Cognitive Sciences* 10: 294–300.

Dugatkin, L. A. 2004. *Principles of Animal Behavior.* New York: W. W. Norton.

Epstein, S. 1994. "Integration of the Cognitive and the Psychodynamic Unconscious." *American Psychologist* 19: 709–24.

Foster, D. J., and M. A. Wilson. 2006. "Reverse Replay of Hippocampal Place Cells during the Awake State." *Nature* 440: 680–83.

Friedman, D. 1998. "Monty Hall's Three Doors: Construction and Deconstruction of a Choice Anomaly." *American Economic Review* 88: 933–46.

Friedrich, J., and A. McGuire. 2010. "Individual Differences in Reasoning Style as a Moderator of the Identifiable Victim Effect." *Social Influence* 5: 182–201.

Greene, J. D. 2013. *Moral Tribes: Emotion, Reason, and the Gap between Us and Them.* New York: Penguin.

Haidt, J. 2001. "The Emotional Dog and Its Rational Tale: A Social Intuitionist Approach to Moral Judgment." *Psychological Review* 108: 814–34.

———. 2007. "The New Synthesis in Moral Psychology." *Science* 316: 998–1002.

Hsee, C. K., and Y. Rottenstreich 2004. "Music, Pandas, and Muggers: On the Affective Psychology of Value." *Journal of Experimental Psychology: General* 133: 23–30.

Ji, D., and M. A. Wilson. 2007. "Coordinated Memory Reply in the Visual Cortex and Hippocampus during Sleep." *Nature Neuroscience* 10: 100–107.
Johnson, A., and A. Redish. 2007. "Neural Ensembles at CA3 Transiently Encode Paths Forward of the Animal at a Decision Point." *Journal of Neuroscience* 27: 12176–89.
Kahneman, D. 2003. "Mapping Bounded Rationality." *American Psychologist* 58: 697–720.
———. 2011. *Thinking, Fast and Slow*. New York: Farrar, Strauss and Giroux.
Kahneman, D., and S. Frederick. 2002. "Representativeness Revisited: Attribute Substitution in Intuitive Judgment." In *Heuristics of Intuitive Judgment: Extensions and Applications*, edited by T. Gilovich, D. Griffin, and D. Kahneman, 49–81. New York: Cambridge University Press.
Kahneman, D., and A. Tversky. 1979. "Prospect Theory: An Analysis of Decision under Risk." *Econometrica* 47: 263–91.
———. 1982. "The Simulation Heuristic." In *Judgment under Uncertainty: Heuristics and Biases*, edited by D. Kahneman, P. Slovic, and A. Tversky, 201–10. New York: Cambridge University Press.
Kahneman, D., and A. Tversky, eds. 2000. *Choices, Values, and Frames*. New York: Cambridge University Press.
Kahneman, D., I. Ritov, and D. Schkade. 1999. "Economic Preferences of Psychological Attitudes: An Analysis of Dollar Responses to Public Issues." *Journal of Risk and Uncertainty* 19: 203–35.
Kogut, T., and I. Ritov. 2004. "The Singularity Effect of Identified Victims in Separate and Joint Evaluations." *Organizational Behavior and Human Decision Processes* 97: 106–16.
———. 2007. "'One of Us': Outstanding Willingness to Help Save a Single Identified Compatriot." *Organizational Behavior and Human Decision Processes* 104: 150–57.
Kolling, N., T. E. J. Behrens, R. B. Mars, and M. F. S. Rushworth. 2012. "Neural Mechanisms of Foraging." *Science* 366: 95–98.
Krebs, J. R., J. T. Erichsen, M. J. Webber, and E. L. Charnov. 1977. "Optimal Prey Selection in the Great Tit (*Parus Major*)." *Animal Behavior* 25: 30–38.
Liley, J., and T. Rakow. 2010. "Probability Estimation in Poker: A Qualified Success for Unaided Judgment." *Journal of Behavioral Decision-Making* 23: 496–526.
Mason, M. F., M. I. Norton, J. D. Van Horn, D. M. Wegner, S. T. Grafteon, and C. N. Macrae. 2007. "Wandering Minds: The Default Network and Stimulus-Independent Thought." *Science* 315: 393–95.
Melis, A. P., B. Hare, and M. Tomasello. 2006. "Chimpanzees Recruit the Best Collaborators." *Science* 311: 1297–300.
Preuschoff, K., P. Bossaerts, and S. Quartz. 2006. "Neural Differentiation of Expected Reward and Risk in Human Subcortical Structures." *Neuron* 51: 381–90.
Raby, C. R., and N. S. Clayton. 2009. "Prospective Cognition in Animals." *Behavioral Processes* 80: 314–24.
Rescorla, R. A. 1988. "Pavlovian Conditioning: It's Not What You Think It Is." *American Psychologist* 43: 151–60.
Reynolds, S. M., and K. C. Berridge. 2008. "Emotional Environments Retune the Valence of Appetitive versus Fearful Functions in Nucleus Accumbens." *Nature Neuroscience* 11: 423–25.
Saffran, J. R., R. N. Aslin, and E. L. Newport. 1996. "Statistical Learning by 8-Month-Old Infants." *Science* 274: 1926–28.

Schultz, W. 2002. "Getting Formal with Dopamine and Reward." *Neuron* 36: 241–63.
Schwartz, N., and G. L. Clore. 1983. "Mood, Misattribution, and Judgments of Well-Being: Informative and Directive Functions of Affective States." *Journal of Personality and Social Psychology* 45: 513–23.
Seligman, M. E. P., P. Railton, R. A. Baumeister, and C. S. Sripada. 2013. "Navigating into the Future or Driven by the Past?" *Perspectives on Psychological Science* 8: 119–41.
Shanks, D. R., R. J. Tunney, and J. D. McCarthy. 2002. "A Re-Examination of Probability Matching and Rational Choice." *Journal of Behavioral Decision Making* 15: 233–50.
Sloman, S. A. 1996. "The Empirical Case for Two Systems of Reasoning." *Psychological Bulletin* 119: 3–22.
Slovic, P., M. Finucane, E. R. Peters, and D. G. MacGregor. 2002. "The Affect Heuristic." In *Heuristics and Biases: The Psychology of Intuitive Judgment*, edited by T. Gilovich, D. Griffin, and D. Kahneman, 397–420. New York: Cambridge University Press.
Small, D. A., and G. Lowenstein. 2003. "Helping the Victim or Helping a Victim: Altruism and Identifiability." *Journal of Risk and Uncertainty* 26: 5–16.
Small, D. A., G. Lowenstein, and P. Slovic. 2007. "Sympathy and Callousness: The Impact of Deliberative Thought on Donations to Identifiable and Statistical Victims." *Organizational Behavior and Human Decision Processes* 102: 143–53.
Suddendorf, T., and M. C. Corballis. 2010. "Behavioural Evidence for Mental Time Travel in Non-human Animals." *Behavioural Brain Research* 215: 292–98.
Taylor, S. E., L. B. Pham, I. D. Rivkin, and D. A. Armor. 1998. "Mental Simulation, Self-Regulation, and Coping." *American Psychologist* 53: 429–39.
Tobler, D. N., J. P. Dougherty, R. J. Dolan, and W. Schultz. 2006. "Reward Value Coding Distinct from Risk Attitude-Related Uncertainty Coding in Human Reward Systems." *Journal of Neurophysiology* 97: 1621–32.
Yarrow, K., P. Brown, and J. W. Krakauer 2009. "Inside the Brain of an Elite Athlete: The Neural Processes That Support High Achievement in Sports." *Nature Reviews: Neuroscience* 10: 585–96.
Zajonc, R. B. 1980. "Preferences Need No Inferences." *American Psychologist* 35: 151–75.
———. 1984. "On the Primacy of Affect." *American Psychologist* 39: 117–23.

PART } II

Ethics and Political Philosophy

3 }

Identified versus Statistical Lives
SOME INTRODUCTORY ISSUES AND ARGUMENTS
Dan W. Brock

In efforts to save lives, the lives that need saving may be either identified or what is typically characterized as statistical. In the case of identified lives, we know the identity of the individual lives at risk and often have information about them, pictures of them, and so forth. So-called statistical lives are lives in a statistical group with a particular risk factor such as high blood pressure. Some intervention such as a medication lowering blood pressure can reduce the deaths in this group—save lives—but we cannot identify which lives are saved and would have been lost without the intervention of the medication.

There are complexities in this very brief characterization of the identified/statistical lives difference, none of which I shall pursue here. I am going to assume that we have enough clarity on the distinction to ask the question that I am interested in: What moral or normative reason could justify giving greater value or weight to saving identified rather than statistical lives? I shall give in the course of my discussion a number of examples that will help to clarify the nature of the difference.

I want to begin with a premise of my discussion, which I call the Principle of the Equal Moral Worth of All Human Lives.[1] This implies that all human persons deserve equal moral concern and respect, as it is sometimes put, and that, all else equal, saving more lives rather than fewer is morally better, produces more moral value, so long as the beneficiaries are chosen fairly. It also implies that all else equal, identified and statistical lives have equal moral value. These are claims about intrinsic moral value. They are compatible with other respects

---

[1] Strictly, this claim should be about the lives of persons, not humans, but for simplicity I use human lives. This difference would be important in many contexts, but so far as I can see it is not important for the identified/statistical issue.

in which the value of lives will differ. For example, different individuals have different economic or other instrumental value; this could be called social value. Given my assumption about the equal moral value of human lives, a defense of the different moral importance of saving identified versus statistical lives requires an argument why this difference matters that is morally compatible with humans' equal moral value. What I will do in this chapter is to examine very briefly seven common arguments that seek to justify giving preference to identified lives over statistical lives. I shall argue that each of these arguments fails. My discussion is introductory in two respects: first, my treatment of each of these arguments is very brief and far from comprehensive; second, there may be other arguments to the same effect, which I do not discuss at all.

1. First Argument: The Rule of Rescue

The Rule of Rescue (RoR) states that if one can save people whose lives are imminently threatened, at reasonable cost or risk to oneself, one has a moral obligation to do so. In the absence of these conditions, one is not always obligated to do so. The RoR is commonly thought to apply to identified, but not to statistical, lives. The RoR was first proposed by Albert Jonsen as a psychological or empirical fact about typical human beings (Jonsen 1986, 172–74). Common examples are miners trapped in a mine collapse, a child who has fallen into a well, or sailors lost at sea. Nearly unlimited efforts with little attention to costs are made to rescue these trapped or lost persons, despite earlier rejection of safety measures that would have saved more persons but were deemed too expensive. Fundraising efforts for serious diseases typically feature pictures or stories of appealing individuals, often children, obviously suffering from those diseases. They tap our compassion and desire to help in a way and to an extent that mere statistics about the problem will not. So the typical human response to seek to help or rescue identified individuals at serious risk is a very basic and deep aspect of human psychology. But as I have formulated the RoR above, it states a moral obligation and is a normative principle. An empirical claim that persons will typically seek, and feel obligated, to rescue identified persons at serious risk of harm is no doubt a largely true generalization about human psychology. But it has no direct moral import and does not constitute any moral argument in defense of the rule of rescue or the preference for identified lives. Humans are generally disposed to favor and benefit family members as opposed to strangers, but that does not morally justify a preference for saving the lives of family members rather than strangers, or that saving the former has greater moral value. What is needed is a moral argument justifying preferring saving identified lives over statistical lives, not merely empirical observations that we act as if there is a moral argument for our doing so. So the rule of rescue, properly understood as an empirical fact of human psychology is no moral argument for preferring saving identified lives over statistical lives.

2. Second Argument: The Moral Importance of Urgency

Identified persons at risk of serious harm are typically in urgent need of help; whereas, statistical victims are typically future lives that will be lost. In many contexts we give priority to those most urgently in need of help, such as triage circumstances in combat or emergency rooms where we must prioritize different patients. Some believe that equity requires priority to the most urgent patients—they are in the greatest need, and in healthcare patients are often prioritized in terms of need (Kamm 1998). One difficulty with this argument is that identified persons do not always have the most urgent conditions. Suppose that from past experience we know that putting in place a highway safety measure, say, installing a traffic light, will immediately result in saving a life in the next six months. These will be statistical lives. We will not know whose life is saved. Alternatively, if we provide a medical intervention anytime in the next year to an identified patient who has a specific but nonurgent medical condition, we will save him from dying a year from now. Here, the needs of the identified persons are the less urgent. But apart from that, why should we think that the more urgent lives at risk should have priority?

Here, it is important to distinguish between temporary and persistent or permanent scarcity. In circumstances of temporary scarcity, such as an accident or disaster that brings more patients to an emergency room than can be treated at once by available staff, urgency is an important criterion in the triaging of patients. The rationale for this practice is that typically, the patients with the most urgent needs will suffer more harm if not treated right away than will those with less urgent needs. If we simplify and just think of patients at risk of death, we will save more lives by attending to the patients with the most urgent needs first. We will have the opportunity to treat those with the less urgent needs later, but we will not have that opportunity to treat and save the patients with the most urgent needs if we do not do so now. Thus, in temporary scarcity, giving moral weight to urgency is a way of maximizing medical benefits or lives saved in the circumstances. No extra priority or value need be given to their lives. The patients with urgent needs have no greater moral importance.

This rationale for giving importance to urgency, however, does not apply in circumstances of persistent scarcity. In persistent scarcity, the degree of scarcity determines how many can be saved or more generally how much medical benefit can be produced with limited resources. Giving significant priority to urgency does not increase overall benefits over time, as it can in temporary scarcity. Instead, it only determines who will be saved, or who will be benefited, when not all can be. It cannot therefore justify saving identified over statistical lives.

The example of organ transplantation demonstrates this most simply and clearly. Suppose there are two patients, Jones, age 60, and Adams, age 40, in need of a life-saving heart or liver transplant; Jones's need is more urgent than Adams's when an organ becomes available, so he gets the transplant and Adams dies. Had Adams's need been more urgent, he would have been saved and Jones would have died. Giving weight to urgency does not enable saving more patients, it only determines who is saved and who is not. Had we given priority to a different criterion such as age, the younger patient, Adams, would have been saved and Jones would have died, but there would be no difference in the number of lives saved. The implication of this for the identified/statistical issue is that even if the most urgent patients are identified and the less urgent are not, this is no moral reason to give more weight to identified than statistical lives on grounds of urgency when prioritizing in persistent scarcity, and much health prioritization is in conditions of persistent resource scarcity.

3. Third Argument: Aggregation

Most people and many theorists prefer giving priority to very large benefits for a few individuals over equally large or larger aggregate benefits consisting of very small benefits for each of a great many more individuals. This is commonly called the aggregation problem, and it was exemplified by the state of Oregon's effort over two decades ago to restructure its Medicaid program. Instead of limiting eligibility for Medicaid to around 60% of the Federal Poverty Level (FPL), its then present level, it proposed to bring eligibility up to the FPL, but limit the services available in the program. To do so, it ranked services by their cost-effectiveness, proposing to begin funding with the most cost-effective services and going down the list until program resources were exhausted, at which point less cost-effective services would not be covered. One result of the initial ranking was that capping teeth was ranked just above appendectomies, despite that fact that the latter was a life-saving intervention. The explanation of this result was that because of the much greater cost of an appendectomy, analysts estimated that over 100 patients needing a tooth capping could be treated for the cost of each appendectomy. If funds ran out after covering tooth cappings, appendectomies would not be covered. This made no sense to most people who considered the list, because their priorities were based principally on one-to-one comparisons, one appendectomy versus one tooth capping, in which case the appendectomy should clearly have priority (Hadorn 1991). The issue was the aggregation problem, whether small benefits to many should have priority over very large benefits to a few if the former were in aggregate larger than the latter (Temkin 2012).

At the time this kind of policy question is addressed, neither the appendectomy nor the dental patients are identified, and after the policy is implemented both groups could be identified, so this does not provide the relevant identified versus statistical comparison. Consider instead a resource allocator who must decide between two programs, one an acute care program that will save 10 patients who will come to the hospital needing care—they will be identified patients when they come to the hospital—and the other, a preventive program that will reduce by an equal or greater number the deaths among a much larger number of 1,000 patients with some risk factor. Those saved by the latter program are and will remain statistical lives—we will never know who the patients are who would have died without the preventive program. On one interpretation, this is still an aggregation problem—10 acute care patients who will be saved versus 1,000 patients who have a reduction in their risk of death of one in a hundred. But on a different interpretation, it is an identified versus statistical comparison—saving 10 identified acute care patients versus saving an equal or somewhat greater number of never identified patients with the prevention program. This is lives saved versus lives saved, not an aggregation problem, and whatever the reason might be for preferring the acute patients, it cannot be moral limits on comparing large benefits to a few versus small benefits to many. Moral limits on aggregation do not favor identified lives.

4. Fourth Argument: Priority to the Worse Off

Many people and many moral theorists believe that in resource prioritization, and particularly in healthcare, we should give at least some priority to the worse off. But who is worse off than identified patients who will imminently die unless they receive treatment? If we consider the example above, of 10 acute care patients versus 1,000 at risk, 10 of whom could be saved by the prevention, it might seem that the acute care patients are worse off—each will die without treatment, whereas in the other group of at-risk patients each has only a 1 in 100 risk of dying without the preventive program. This is why it seems that the acute patients are clearly worse off. But the harm to each of the 10 statistical patients who will die without the prevention program, even if we can never know their identity, is the same as that to the acute patients without treatment—death. So the comparison is 10 deaths of acute patients versus 10 deaths of patients who can be saved by prevention. The only difference is that the latter are not identified; there is no difference between the two groups in how worse off their members are. Priority to the worse off does not favor either group.

Interestingly, if reducing a risk that would not have eventuated in harm to most of those at risk, but at a time when who they are is not known, is a benefit to those whose risk is reduced, then the prevention alternative might be thought to produce a greater benefit even if it only saves 10 statistical lives, the same number as the acute treatment saves. That is because it produces the ex ante benefit of elimination of a 1 in 100 risk of death for all those in the at-risk group, plus the benefit of saving the 10 statistical lives who without it would have died. The issue here is whether eliminating an ex ante risk that would later turn out ex post not to eventuate is a benefit, and whether reducing that risk ex ante before it would ex post either eventuate or not eventuate is a benefit. Whatever one's assessment of this issue, priority for the worse off seems not to provide a basis for favoring identified over statistical lives.

5. Fifth Argument: Uncertainty

Particularly when the statistical lives are lives saved by prevention programs, it might be thought that uncertainty provides a reason for favoring identified lives. As with some of the other arguments considered above, there are two problems with this argument. First, before we act we can only assess the expected number of identified lives that would be saved by the acute intervention versus the expected number of statistical lives that would be saved by the prevention intervention. There may be little uncertainty about whether the identified acute patients will be saved with treatment. On the other hand, if the prevention program's effects will be some 20 years hence, many factors may intervene to change and reduce the number of lives that that program will save—those at risk may die from other causes, cures may be developed that will save them instead, and so forth. But this uncertainty should already have been taken account of in estimating the expected identified lives that will be saved by the respective interventions. It would double count the uncertainty to give more importance to the identified lives on grounds that they are more certain, after having already taken that into account at the point of estimating the expected lives each intervention will save. This would not, however, necessarily be true. Some people might be risk-averse in lives saved, so would value saving 10 for sure over a fifty-fifty gamble of saving zero or 20 lives, even though both have the same "expectation." But then this risk aversion is in need of justification.

The other difficulty with the uncertainty argument is that uncertainty does not always map onto the identified/statistical difference as I assumed it did in the example above. It may be highly uncertain that acute care interventions will succeed with identified patients in imminent risk of harm or death; for example, such interventions may have rarely worked with similar patients in the past. But prevention programs that will save only statistical lives may be highly certain to save those lives, though the identity of the lives remains unknown, since they have nearly always worked so in the past. Uncertainty may sometimes be greater with identified lives at risk.

6. Sixth Argument: Temporal Discounting

Many prevention interventions such as changes in unhealthy behavior or vaccination programs benefit statistical patients but benefit statistical patients only years after the intervention. Acute care interventions typically benefit identified patients in the present. In assessing benefits and costs for cost-effectiveness analyses, it is standard practice to apply a temporal discount rate to them in the range of 3% to 5% (Gold et al. 1996). This means, for example, that an intervention that saves 100 lives now has significantly greater value than an alternative intervention that will save 100 lives 20 years from now. Since acute care interventions for identified patients typically save these identified lives in the near future, while many preventive interventions for statistical patients only save lives in the more distant future, this could be a basis for assigning more value to identified lives. As with many of the previous arguments, this application of discounting will not always map onto the identified/statistical distinction, for example, if both the acute and preventive interventions produce their benefits in the present. But that is not the main difficulty with this argument.

The crucial issue is whether health benefits, such as saving lives, should be discounted in this way. There is no controversy that monetary costs and benefits should be discounted for familiar reasons—if the costs of a health program can be postponed, its funding requires fewer current dollars, and likewise if monetary benefits are received now instead of later they can be invested in the meantime. But why should health benefits such as lives saved be discounted? Doing so means that we should prefer and value saving 100 lives now rather than 120 lives in 20 years, when all else is equal—the 120 lives discounted at 3% are less than the 100 lives now. But the principle of the equal value of human lives implies that a life today is of no more value than a life in 20 years—temporal discounting of lives violates that principle (Broome 1994).

This issue has great practical importance. Since prevention programs often produce their benefits significantly into the future, while acute care programs do so largely in the present, discounting will significantly disadvantage prevention programs when their cost-effectiveness is compared with acute care programs. This is one reason for the common observation of the apparent underfunding for prevention programs. The implications of discounting are most implausible in the context of many environmental issues. The risks of alternatives for disposing of nuclear waste, for example, may not eventuate for several hundred years. At a 5% discount rate, Derek Parfit has calculated that one life today has roughly the same value as a billion lives in 400 years. That cannot be a morally acceptable implication.

7. Seventh Argument: Special Relationships

Many people believe that it is morally justified, or at least morally permissible, to give special importance to those with whom we stand in special relationships, such as family members or close friends. It is permissible to save one's spouse or child even at the cost of not being able to save two strangers. Many moral theorists support this common view as well (Williams 1973; Scheffler 1992). Consequentialists typically reject this position, but it is one of a number of serious conflicts between consequentialism and common morality. Supporters of the special-relationships view will have to say how much additional importance can justifiably be given to which relationships, since morality must place some limits on their special importance, but this is not the central difficulty in applying this view to the identified/statistical lives issue. As earlier, the distinction between those in special relationships versus those who are not (such as strangers) fails to map onto the identified versus statistical lives distinction. An identified person whose life is at risk and needs to be saved may be a stranger, and the special relationship may exist with a group from which statistical lives saved would come, such as coworkers, fellow countrymen, and so forth.

8. Conclusion So Far

Each of the arguments I have considered above aims to show that the distinction between identified and statistical lives is in itself morally significant; more specifically, that saving identified lives is morally more valuable than saving statistical lives. I have argued that there are two sorts of difficulties with these defenses of the identified/statistical distinction, at least one (and usually both) of which undermine that defense. The first difficulty is that these other distinctions, such as the worse off versus the better off, fail always to map onto the identified versus statistical distinction. So these arguments could at most show that the identified/statistical distinction is sometimes morally significant when it correlates with other morally significant differences, but not in itself. The second difficulty is that these arguments often appeal to other distinctions, such as the psychological salience of the life being identified or the urgency of the need for help. Because they are not themselves morally significant, they cannot support the intrinsic moral significance of the identified/statistical difference.

9. A Different Kind of Argument

There is a different kind of argument relevant here that does not reject the principle of the equal moral value of human lives. So it does not appeal to any argument of the sort I have been considering that seeks to establish that identified lives, and so saving them, are in themselves morally of more value than statistical lives. Instead, this argument claims that at least in many circumstances, giving higher priority or preference to identified over statistical lives produces greater overall value, despite the fact that the lives are identified rather than statistical is not in itself morally significant. Here are three examples of plausible arguments of this sort. It seems to be a fact that donors will give more resources for HIV treatment of identified patients than prevention of HIV and AIDS in statistical patients. There may be different reasons for this, such as the psychological motivation of seeing pictures or hearing the stories of the patients in need of treatment. But whatever the reasons, saving more lives is, all other things equal, better than saving fewer. If giving priority to identified lives in need of treatment rather than statistical lives that could be saved by prevention enables us to save more lives, then it can be morally justified and is not in conflict with the equal moral value of all human life. A second example: if we have to stand by and not save identified imperiled individuals because our efforts and resources could be used instead for prevention efforts that would save more statistical lives, this could be dehumanizing and eroding of important moral motivation and compassion for others, with bad effects on balance for preserving human life. A third example: other people get utility from the rescue of imperiled individuals besides the individuals themselves who are rescued; cases of widely publicized life-saving—the girl in the well—are examples of this. Each of these examples rests on the empirical claim that giving greater priority to identified lives in the specified circumstances either enables the saving of more lives, or produces more overall value. I have no objection to these kinds of arguments, so long as there is evidence for the empirical claims on which they depend. And this is also how some of the arguments that I have considered above should be interpreted. When, but only when, a morally important principle like priority to the worse off maps onto the identified/statistical difference, then the identified/statistical difference is morally important—but that is because of the other principle—in this case, priority to the worse off—not the difference between identified and statistical lives.

References

Broome, J. 1994. "Discounting the Future." *Philosophy and Public Affairs* 23: 128–56. Reprinted in *Ethics Out of Economics* (Cambridge: Cambridge University Press, 1999), 44–67.
Gold, M. R., et al. 1996. *Cost-Effectiveness in Health and Medicine*. New York: Oxford University Press.
Hadorn, D. C. 1991. "Setting Health Care Priorities in Oregon: Cost-Effectiveness Meets the Rule of Rescue." *Journal of the American Medical Association* 265 (17): 2218–25.

Jonsen, A. R. 1986. "Bentham in a Box: Technology Assessment and Health Care Allocation." *Law, Medicine and Health Care* 14 (3–4): 172–74.

Kamm, F. M. 1998. *Morality/Mortality: Death and Whom to Save from It*. Oxford: Oxford University Press.

Scheffler, Samuel. 1992. "Prerogatives without Restrictions." *Philosophical Perspectives* 6: 377–97.

Temkin, Larry S. 2012. *Rethinking the Good: Moral Ideals and the Nature of Practical Reasoning*. New York: Oxford University Press.

Williams, B. 1973. "A Critique of Utilitarianism." In *Utilitarianism: For and Against*, edited by B. Williams and J. J. C. Smart, 77–150. Cambridge: Cambridge University Press.

4 }

Welfarism, Equity, and the Choice between Statistical and Identified Victims

Matthew D. Adler

1. Introduction and Setup

Should policymakers give priority to saving "identified" as opposed to "statistical" victims? Such priority is embodied in the following principle, denoted PSIV for short. By "status quo," here and throughout the chapter, I mean governmental inaction: the policy choice of doing nothing.

Priority for Saving Identified Victims (PSIV)
Assume that one person (the "identified victim") would die prematurely, for certain, if government were to leave in place the status quo. There are two or more other persons (the "statistical victims") who would each be at nonzero risk of dying prematurely if government were to leave in place the status quo, and these risks sum to 1. Assume, moreover, that one policy, with certainty, saves the first person from premature death—and has no effect on other individuals. A second policy reduces the risk of premature death of each person in the second group to zero—again, with no effect on other individuals. (Note that, under these assumptions, each policy reduces the number of expected premature deaths by one.)[1]

---

[1] The first policy changes the identified victim's risk of dying from 1 to 0, and this clearly reduces the expected number of premature deaths by one. The second policy also (perhaps less obviously) reduces the expected number of premature deaths by one. Why? In general, the sum of the changes in individuals' probabilities of premature death—which here, by construction, is –1—is just the change in the expected number of premature deaths. This in turn follows from a theorem of probability calculus, namely that the sum of the expected values of a collection of random variables is the expected value of the sum of those random variables. Think of each person in the population as corresponding to a random variable with value 1 if she dies prematurely and 0 if she lives. Her probability of premature death is just the expected value of this random variable, and the expected number of premature deaths just the expected sum of these random variables across the population.

If all this is true, and known to government, and government can only choose one of the two policies, it should choose the first.

Is PSIV a normatively attractive principle? Should we endorse or reject it?

PSIV, as just formulated, concerns the risk of death. Discussions of priority for identified victims often occur in the context of health and safety regulation, where fatality risks are paramount. A priority with respect to the harm of death might generalize to nonfatal harms. But it is not obvious that it would thus generalize—even for welfarists.[2] I thus take a first stab at the problem of priority by focusing on the harm of death. In the analysis to follow, therefore, the term "death" is implied where not explicit: "risk" mean risk of death, "victim" someone who dies or might die, and so on.

PSIV, as just formulated, concerns someone who is an identified victim in the strongest possible sense. Absent government intervention, she is certain to die. If such a victim takes priority, then wouldn't it also be true that government should target risk reduction to persons at high risk of premature death, even if they are not certain to die? Below, in the course of analyzing PSIV, I will discuss an axiom of "Risk Transfer," which does entail that reducing someone's risk of premature death by a certain amount is better than reducing someone else's risk by the same amount, if the first individual starts out at higher risk of death than the second and they are otherwise identical.

However, it is not obvious—even for welfarists—that someone who accepts PSIV should accept Risk Transfer. As we shall see below, Risk Transfer plus an additional axiom logically implies PSIV; but it is possible to endorse PSIV while rejecting Risk Transfer. I organize and focus my analysis by making the status of PSIV, specifically, the central question of the chapter.

The problem of statistical versus identified victims is presented most clearly by ignoring nonrisk differences between these groups. Assume that all individuals at risk of dying prematurely (either in the status quo or given some other policy choice) are identical with respect to income, health, happiness, and all other welfare-relevant nonrisk attributes (including their preferences); and that the different risk-reduction policies under consideration do not change these attributes among this group of individuals. I will refer to this as the "ceteris paribus" premise. And I will refer to the principle PSIV, in the case where the ceteris paribus premise holds true, as the "ceteris paribus" PSIV.

The ceteris paribus PSIV is a less ambitious and controversial principle than one that says government should give priority to saving identified victims even

---

[2] Within the context of the "social welfare function" (SWF) framework, as elaborated below, a priority for identified victims flows from the ex ante Pigou-Dalton principle—which itself concerns the distribution of expected utility and does not differentiate between death and other harms. By contrast, under cost-benefit analysis (CBA), again as elaborated below, such priority is the upshot of a standard model for calculating the "value of statistical life," plus a particular methodology for calculating individuals' monetary equivalents. It is not obvious whether CBA for nonfatal harms would embody a parallel priority.

if statistical victims are worse off with respect to nonrisk attributes. And it will be the ceteris paribus PSIV principle that this chapter generally addresses—dropping the phrase "ceteris paribus," which is henceforth implied.

"Should" questions might be moral questions, or questions about "should" in some nonmoral sense. This chapter focuses on the moral status of saving identified versus statistical victims. (Locutions such as "saving identified versus statistical victims" are used as synonyms for conformity with PSIV.) And the chapter discusses the moral status of PSIV through the lens of *welfarism*. Welfarism (as here understood) is a class of moral views, having in common the feature that they morally evaluate choices in light of the associated distributions of individual well-being.

More precisely, let W_1 be a group of outcomes homogeneous with respect to individual well-being: any particular individual's well-being is the same regardless of which outcome within W_1 occurs. W_2 is another such group, W_3 yet another. Any given choice a (e.g., a governmental policy choice) will have a probability $p_1(a)$ of producing some outcome within W_1, a probability $p_2(a)$ of producing some outcome within W_2, a probability $p_3(a)$ of producing some outcome within W_3, and so on. Then welfarists say that the moral ranking of a set of choices $\{a, a^*, \ldots\}$ just depends on these probabilities.[3] Considerations other than individual well-being—for example, whether one choice violates a deontological side-constraint—are irrelevant.

It might be thought that welfarists are committed to ranking policies in light of expected premature deaths—at least where the individuals whose fatality risks are affected by the policies are otherwise identical—and therefore that welfarism displays no preference for saving identified victims.[4] This thought is doubly untrue—as we shall see. First, there are versions of welfarism

---

[3] A standard definition of welfarism is in terms of "supervenience": if each person is just as well off in outcome x as she is in outcome y, the two outcomes are equally good. The definition in the text is essentially the same as the standard definition—but adapted to the context of ranking choices with uncertain outcomes. Note that the definition in the text is framed in terms of intrapersonal comparisons, and does not presuppose that well-being is also interpersonally comparable. The definition is thus broad enough that CBA (using equivalent variations) counts as "welfarist." (On the distinction between equivalent and compensating variations, see Adler, Hammitt and Treich 2014; appendix. CBA with compensating variations turns out not to be 'welfarist' as just defined, for technical reasons not worth elaborating here, but for completeness both versions of CBA will be discussed below.) The definition in the text is also broad enough to encompass both "ex post" and "ex ante" approaches to applying an SWF under conditions of uncertainty, as elaborated below. Note, finally, that the definition is framed in terms of "outcomes" but does not entail the more specific axiom of "Consequentialism"—which will be pivotal to the analysis below and which textbook CBA as well as one version of the SWF approach violates.

[4] Ranking policies in light of expected premature deaths clearly violates PSIV, as formulated here. Assume that, in the status quo, one individual is certain to die prematurely. Policy P reduces her risk of premature death to 0 and has no other effect. There is also a group of two or more persons each of whom has a nonzero risk of premature death, and whose cumulative risk of premature death is 1. Policy P^* reduces their risks to 0 and has no other effect. Then P and P^* have the same number of expected premature deaths, but PSIV prefers P.

that satisfy PSIV. Second, there are important variants of welfarism that reject PSIV, but do not rank policies in light of expected deaths (even where all individuals are identical except in their fatality risks).

Welfarists, of course, should care about welfarism's verdict regarding identified versus statistical lives. But so should welfarism's critics. Debates between welfarists and nonwelfarists should be undertaken with an appreciation of the nuances of the different moral frameworks on offer.

The chapter discusses two welfarist frameworks: cost-benefit analysis (CBA) and the social welfare function (SWF). CBA is now the dominant policy-analysis methodology employed by the US government, and a methodology increasingly used abroad. Surprisingly, one version of the textbook approach to CBA actually does prefer saving identified lives. However, CBA understood as a moral framework is quite problematic, for reasons well rehearsed in the scholarly literature. (On CBA, see generally Adler 2012, 86–114, and sources cited therein; Adler and Posner 2006.)

The SWF framework is also welfarist, but differs from CBA in using interpersonally comparable utilities, rather than money, as the scale for measuring individual well-being. One popular SWF is "utilitarian." A different type of SWF might be termed "equity" or "fairness" regarding. Under conditions of uncertainty, the utilitarian SWF can be applied in an "ex ante" or "ex post" manner. Similarly, we can differentiate between "ex ante" and "ex post" methodologies for applying an equity-regarding SWF under uncertainty. (On SWFs, see generally Adler 2012, especially chs. 2, 5, 7, and sources cited therein; Bossert and Weymark 2004.)

This yields four specifications of the SWF approach, all worth consideration. As we shall see, ex ante and ex post utilitarianism violate PSIV, as does an ex post equity-regarding approach. However, the ex ante equity-regarding approach does give priority to saving identified victims. Ex ante utilitarianism, ex post utilitarianism, and the ex post equity-regarding approach all satisfy a principle I shall term *Consequentialism*, which is logically incompatible with PSIV. By contrast, the ex ante approach satisfies PSIV in virtue of satisfying the *Ex Ante Pigou-Dalton Principle*.

What emerges from this analysis is that the problem of statistical versus identified lives cannot be settled at the level of welfarism, nor as part of the debate about CBA, nor even by rejecting utilitarianism. Ex ante and ex post equity-regarding approaches concur in embracing welfarism, rejecting CBA, and embracing a concern for an equitable distribution of well-being (thus rejecting utilitarianism). Their disagreement concerns a much more subtle problem: equity-regarding policy choice under conditions of uncertainty.

The analysis is undertaken using a simple model, the formal details of which are presented in an appendix, and which is discussed informally in the main text. The policymaker faces a set of policy choices, including the status quo choice of inaction. There are different possible "states of the world" (for short, "states") that have probabilities summing to 1; and a fixed population of individuals. As in the standard representation of choice under uncertainty originating with Leonard Savage, the combination of a choice and a state yields an outcome: a (more or less) complete description of a final allocation of welfare-relevant characteristics among the individuals. Thus, a "state" should be understood as a combination of background causal factors sufficient to determine—in combination with the policymaker's choice—which outcome will occur. (See Adler 2012, 481–90.)

In the model employed here, there is a current period (some slice of time that includes the present), and each individual's attributes in a given outcome include the following: whether she dies during the current period, or survives to die at a later time; her income in the current period; and all other attributes (her current nonincome attributes, her past attributes, and her future attributes conditional on surviving the current period).

It must be remembered that everyone dies eventually; and that government "saves" individuals, statistical or identified, not by shielding them entirely from death, but rather by preventing them from dying earlier rather than later. The relevant certainties, risks, and risk reductions concern premature death. In our simple model, premature death equals death during the current period.[5] Given a particular choice (whether a policy intervention by government, or the status quo choice of policy inaction), someone's probability of dying during the current period is the sum of the probability of those states of the world whose outcomes (as a result of that choice) are such that the individual dies during the current period. So as to avoid repetition, the term "premature" or "in the current period" is often dropped below.

In this model, all probabilities are known to government: there is no disjunction between a given person's "real"[6] probability of death, and the probability that governmental officials believe to be her death probability. An "identified" victim, therefore, is someone whose real status quo risk of dying is 1 and is believed by the policymaker to face this risk. A "statistical victim" is someone whose real status quo risk of dying is less than 1 and greater than 0. In a richer model, someone might have a real death risk of 1, but be a "statistical" victim in the sense that no one knows her to have this risk.

This model will be used as a test bed for the ceteris paribus PSIV. We therefore assume that, in all outcomes (whether possible outcomes of the status quo, or of some policy intervention) all individuals have the very same current

---

[5] Thus, each individual has a determinate life-span (the same in every state), conditional on surviving the current period.

[6] "Real" means morally relevant. What the morally relevant probabilities are (objective "chances," epistemically reasonable degrees of belief, etc.) is a matter of moral dispute. My analysis is agnostic on the question.

income, and the very same nonincome attributes except for surviving or perishing during the current period. Individuals also have the same preferences.[7] In the status quo, individuals may differ with respect to their risk of death, but are otherwise identical; and policies reduce risk for some individuals, but leave them otherwise identical.

One aspect of the ceteris paribus assumption, important to note, is that individuals at higher risk of death are assumed not to be at a higher level of anxiety or fear because of this risk. In reality, of course, risk levels do correlate with fear, anxiety, and other affects. But then government has a reason quite apart from risk- or death-reduction to prioritize certain victims, a reason that welfarists of all stripes could approve—reducing fear or other welfare-reducing emotional states (Adler 2004). The question, here, is how the patterns of individuals' risks—holding constant everything else that determines individual well-being, including emotions or other welfare-relevant mental states—shape the moral considerations bearing on governmental policy choice.[8]

It might be supposed that being at higher risk of premature death is a welfare setback, independent of premature death actually occurring, and independent of fears or any other mental setbacks associated with the risk. Assume that in the status quo, Ariel (unbeknownst to her) had a high risk of premature death, while Benjamin (unbeknownst to him) had a low risk. Government does nothing; the risks are not realized and neither dies prematurely (Ariel is lucky!); and outcome x results, with Ariel and Benjamin living identical lifespans, having the same income level, being equally healthy and happy, and otherwise having equally good lives except that Ariel was at higher risk, Benjamin at lower risk. Is Ariel thereby worse off than Benjamin in outcome x? I assume not. The realized goodness of lives—the level of well-being associated with a given person in a given final outcome—depends upon that person's physical, mental, social, and other attributes in that outcome; but being at risk, as such, independent of its impact on other attributes, does not change the level of realized well-being.[9]

---

[7] Under CBA, monetary equivalents are defined in terms of individuals' preferences. In general, CBA does not require homogeneity of preferences. However, the simple model used in the appendix (reflecting the ceteris paribus assumption) does presuppose preference homogeneity.

[8] On some theories of well-being, the sheer knowledge of being at higher risk—apart from increased fear or other negative emotions—can reduce individual well-being. If the reader finds such a view plausible, she should imagine that the individuals at various risk levels in the status quo, and who might be benefited by governmental intervention, do not even know about these risks (let alone fear them). Government knows the risks, but the beneficiaries do not. Again, this simplifying assumption, surely unrealistic, is designed to sharpen moral reflection by clarifying whether those at high risk have a moral priority as such.

[9] Defending the premise is well beyond the scope of this chapter. I have elsewhere defended a view of well-being such that someone's welfare depends upon her well-informed, rational, and self-interested preferences. Such a view allows for an individual to be harmed by events outside her body or mind—for example, being betrayed by a spouse (Adler 2012, ch. 3; Adler 2013). If Felix, whom Sylvia wrongly believes to be her friend, imposes a risk upon Sylvia out of contempt—say, by playing Russian roulette

TABLE 4.1 } A Mortality Matrix

	States			Survival Probability
Individuals	$s; \pi(s) = .2$	$s^*; \pi(s^*) = .5$	$s^{**}; \pi(s^{**}) = .3$	
Able	1	0	1	.5
Baker	1	1	0	.7
Charlie	0	0	1	.3

Given the ceteris paribus assumption, plus the premise just stated, the ranking of policy choices by CBA, by the SWF approach, or for that matter by any other welfarist methodology is solely a function of the *morality matrices* associated with these choices, plus the fixed list (whatever it may be) of identical nonrisk attributes for all individuals. The mortality matrix for a given choice displays, for each individual, whether she survives the current period or dies prematurely in each possible state—with 1 denoting survival and 0 death. See Table 4.1.

2. Cost-Benefit Analysis

The textbook version of CBA values fatality risk reductions (like all other changes) by summing monetary equivalents, calculated in one of two ways: (1) an individual's monetary equivalent for a policy that reduces her risk by Δp[10] is the amount Δc such that, if her income in all possible policy outcomes were reduced by Δc, she would be indifferent between the policy and the status quo; (2) an individual's monetary equivalent for a policy that reduces her risk by Δp is the amount $\Delta c'$ such that, if her income in all possible status quo outcomes were increased by $\Delta c'$, she would be indifferent between the status quo and the policy.

As Δp approaches zero, the ratio between the individual's monetary equivalent (calculated either way) and Δp converges to a number. This number is known as the individual's "value of statistical life" (VSL)—a terrible but

---

with Sylvia as victim while she sleeps—then this event arguably does make Sylvia's life worse even if she never learns of it. The premise does not deny this; it just says that being put at risk must be associated with something else (fear, betrayal, false beliefs—what these would need to be is a matter for further discussion) to be an outcome harm.

Also, it needs to be stressed that the premise does not deny the relevance of risks to policy choices. That would be absurd. If the decision-maker is uncertain about which outcome would occur as a result of her choice, she of course needs to attend to the probabilities of the outcomes that she takes to be possible. The point, rather, is that the comparative goodness or badness of outcomes for individual well-being is not itself a matter of the probabilities leading to them. Which action should be chosen is a function of the probabilities of the outcomes, plus the outcomes, with outcomes themselves characterized independently of the probabilities.

[10] Throughout this discussion the quantity Δp is assumed to be positive.

now-standard term. The VSL_i for a given individual i is the limit of her trade-off rate between income and risk reduction, as the risk reduction becomes smaller and smaller. Individual i's monetary equivalent (Δc or $\Delta c'$) for a policy that reduces her risk by Δp is approximately equal to Δp multiplied by VSL_i—with this approximation becoming better and better as Δp approaches zero. (On VSL and CBA for risk reduction, see generally Adler, Hammitt, and Treich 2014, and sources cited therein.)

Another way to think of VSL_i is that this is the conversion factor that translates a small risk change for individual i into a dollar equivalent. For example, if we specify a 1 in 1,000,000 risk change as one unit, and VSL_i is $6/unit, then individual i's monetary equivalent for a 1 in 100,000 change in her probability of dying is $60.

VSL_i depends upon individual i's status quo income; her status quo fatality risk; and her other status quo attributes. In general, because individuals vary in these attributes, VSL can vary as well. In the model at hand, with the ceteris paribus assumption adopted and everything but fatality risk identical among individuals, VSL will still vary. As shown in the appendix, VSL increases with fatality risk. If i has a higher status quo fatality risk than j, then VSL_i is greater than VSL_j. This means that individual i has a greater monetary equivalent for a given reduction in status quo risk, as compared to individual j, if the risk reduction is sufficiently small. Intuitively, because current income is less useful to someone who dies during the current period, individual i's expected marginal utility of income is lower than j's, and individual i is willing to sacrifice more income for a risk reduction than j.[11] This effect is known in the literature as the "dead anyway" effect.

Because VSL increases with fatality risk, it follows immediately that CBA has the following feature: If i has a greater status quo risk of dying than j, then CBA will disprefer the status quo to a policy that reduces i's status quo risk by Δp and increases j's status quo risk by Δp, leaving everyone else's risk unchanged—at least if Δp is sufficiently small (close to zero). In short, CBA necessarily prefers a sufficiently small risk transfer from those with a higher status quo risk of dying, to those with a lower such risk.

What if Δp is larger? And what if there is a transfer of risk Δp—from someone at higher risk of dying to someone at lower risk—that occurs by

---

[11] While the ceteris paribus assumption means that individuals have identical nonrisk characteristics (including income) in all outcomes with nonzero probability—both status quo outcomes and outcomes of the alternative policies being considered—we can still ascertain what an individual's expected utility would be if his income were varied along with fatality risk.

The intuition that an individual's current income has less utility and marginal utility if the individual dies during the current period (as per the simple model of VSL in the appendix) holds good only if the individual's expenditure plan for the income is independent of his perceived risk of dying. Arguably, "bucket list" expenditures in the shadow of death might have a very large impact on well-being. But the model is too simple to capture this possibility.

moving from one policy to a second, where neither policy is the status quo? The axiom of Risk Transfer addresses these cases—articulating a general priority for individuals at higher risk of dying.

Risk Transfer
Imagine that individual i has a higher fatality risk with policy a than individual j. (Policy a can be the status quo or any other policy choice.) As compared to policy a, policy b reduces individual i's risk by Δp and increases individual j's risk by the same amount, and moreover the risk gap between them decreases. Finally, everyone else's fatality risk is the same with both policies. Then, if individuals are identical with respect to nonrisk attributes (the ceteris paribus assumption holds), policy b is a better policy than a.

It turns out that CBA does not satisfy Risk Transfer (see appendix; Adler, Hammitt, and Treich 2014). The reason, in a nutshell, is that the expected marginal utility of income is determined not only by risk level but also by income level. This second determinant comes into play for large risk transfers, or transfers involving two policies neither of which is the status quo, even where individuals have the same income. To get an intuitive sense why, consider the following. If Sebastian in the status quo is at a given income and survival probability (c, p) and a policy changes his survival probability by a large amount Δp^*, then Sebastian's money equivalent for Δp^* is equal to the sum of his money equivalents $(\Delta c_0 + \Delta c_1 + \cdots + \Delta c_M)$ for the series of small changes $\Delta p_0 + \Delta p_1 + \cdots + \Delta p_M = \Delta p^*$—with Δc_1 his money equivalent for the change Δp_1 at status quo income changed by Δc_0, Δc_2 his money equivalent for the change Δp_2 at status quo income changed by $\Delta c_0 + \Delta c_1$, and so forth. Note now that the conversion factor translating Δp_1 into Δc_1 will be determined by the expected marginal utility of income not at original income c, but at c changed by Δc_0. Similarly, the conversion factor translating Δp_2 into Δc_2 will be determined by the expected marginal utility of income not at original income c, but at c changed by $\Delta c_0 + \Delta c_1$—and so on.

It might be conjectured that CBA, because it violates Risk Transfer, also violates PSIV. Interestingly, this is not true. It can be shown that the second textbook version of CBA described above—the version that calculates monetary equivalents as changes to status quo income—does in fact satisfy PSIV (see appendix). Why? If an increase in current status quo income of the person sure to die prematurely in the status quo makes no difference to her lifetime well-being, then her money equivalent for being saved is infinite—while each statistical victim has a finite equivalent for elimination of his status quo risk of death. Conversely, if an increase in the identified victim's current status quo income does make a well-being difference, it can be shown that the increase required to make her as well off as she would be if saved (with no change to her income) is greater than the sum of the amounts required to make the statistical victims equally well off as between receiving those amounts (with no change to their risks) and having the risks eliminated (with no change to their incomes).

CBA in governmental practice differs from the textbook versions by suppressing variation in monetary equivalents for risk reduction. At least in the United States, official bodies tend to assume that all individuals have the same VSL, regardless of differences in income, status quo risk of dying, or other attributes. (Robinson 2007.) The monetized benefit of any individual's risk reduction Δp is simply Δp multiplied by this constant value—a population average VSL, estimated to be in the range of \$7 million. CBA in this form embodies no preference for saving identified victims. The total monetized risk-reduction benefit of a given policy is just its reduction in expected deaths (as compared to the status quo) multiplied by the population average VSL. Thus, in the case where the ceteris paribus assumption is adopted, the ranking of policies by governmental CBA is just a function of their expected number of premature deaths.

In sum, CBA's treatment of risk reduction turns out to be quite complex. In the textbook versions, it approves a small risk transfer that reduces by Δp the status quo risk of someone at higher risk of dying, and increases by Δp the status quo risk of someone with the same income but at lower risk of dying. Neither textbook version satisfies a more general axiom of Risk Transfer, but one textbook version of CBA turns out to satisfy PSIV. Governmental practice, using a constant VSL, is wholly insensitive to the risk levels of those who benefit from risk-reducing policies—focusing just on the cumulative reduction, that is, the decrease in expected premature deaths.

It is intellectually interesting to note that one version of CBA, if not the approach actually used in governmental practice, embodies a preference for saving identified lives. But CBA (whatever version) is hardly a sure guide to moral requirements—even for welfarists. At best CBA is a kind of rough, fallible, proxy for a utilitarian SWF: a decision procedure, rather than a criterion of moral goodness. It would be wrongheaded to make inferences about the moral status of PSIV from the fact that CBA in some version endorses, or fails to endorse, that principle.

3. Social Welfare Functions

The SWF approach grows out of theoretical welfare economics and is employed in various areas of economic research. The approach also has many links to moral philosophy.

Leaving aside uncertainty for the moment, SWFs can be differentiated by how they rank outcomes. Any given outcome is mapped onto a list ("vector") of utility numbers, one for each member of the population, representing the well-being level of that individual in that outcome. An SWF is simply some transitive rule for ranking these utility vectors from best to worst. Many such rules are possible. Via axiomatic analysis, we can narrow down the set of plausible such rules (see Adler 2012, ch. 5).

Two very plausible principles are Anonymity and the Pareto principle. Anonymity says that if two outcomes are associated with utility vectors that are just rearrangements of each other—if the two have the same pattern of utility and differ simply in which particular individuals are at which utility levels—the two are equally good. The Pareto principle says that if each person's utility level in one outcome is at least as high as in a second outcome, with some individuals having strictly greater utility in the first outcome, the first outcome is better.

The *utilitarian* SWF uses a simple additive rule: Utility vectors are ranked by simple summation of their component numbers. The utilitarian SWF does satisfy Anonymity and the Pareto principle. However, utilitarianism is notoriously insensitive to the *fair distribution* of well-being. As between two outcomes with the same total amount of well-being, utilitarianism is indifferent between the two, even if the distribution of well-being is perfectly equal in the first and highly unequal in the second.

A concern for fair/equitable distribution is captured, axiomatically, in the Pigou-Dalton principle (for outcomes). This principle says: If in one outcome some individual has less utility than a second, and we change the outcome so that the first individual's utility is increased by some amount, the second individual's is reduced by the very same amount, this change shrinks the utility gap between the two, and no one else is affected, this change is a moral improvement. Many different kinds of nonutilitarian SWFs satisfy the Pigou-Dalton principle (for outcomes) as well as Anonymity and the Pareto principle. I shall term this family of SWFs *equity-regarding* SWFs.

In other scholarship, I have argued for a *prioritarian* SWF, which represents one kind of equity-regarding SWF (Adler 2012, ch. 5). For purposes of PSIV, the distinction between prioritarian and nonprioritarian equity-regarding SWFs is not important, and so the analysis in this chapter shall consider equity-regarding SWFs as a group.

Turning now to uncertainty, a given policy (or the status quo) is seen by the SWF framework as a probability distribution over utility vectors, and a resultant vector of individual expected utilities (on SWFs under uncertainty, see Adler 2012 ch. 7). Any particular SWF can now be applied to rank policies in two ways: (1) an "ex post" manner, namely, by assigning a number to each policy equaling the expected value of the SWF; or (2) an "ex ante" manner, namely by applying the SWF to each policy's vector of individual expected utilities.[12]

---

[12] A yet more complicated possibility is a mixture of ex post and ex ante (Adler 2012, 516 n. 74; Mongin and Pivato, forthcoming). This is ignored here.

TABLE 4.2 } Ex Post versus Ex Ante

Individuals	States		Expected Utility
	$s: \pi(s) = .5$	$s^*: \pi(s^*) = .5$	
Able	100	16	58
Baker	9	25	17
Value of SWF in each state	$\sqrt{100} + \sqrt{9} = 13$	$\sqrt{16} + \sqrt{25} = 9$	

Note: The entry in each cell is the individual's utility in that state. Let the SWF be the sum of the square root of individual utilities. The ex post approach assigns this policy the expected value of the SWF, i.e., $(.5)13 + (.5)9 = 11$. The ex ante approach applies the SWF to the vector of expected utilities, i.e., $\sqrt{58} + \sqrt{17} = 11.74$.

(See appendix for a more formal definition.) These approaches are illustrated in Table 4.2.

Combining the "ex post"/"ex ante" distinction with the two types of SWF under consideration, utilitarian and equity-regarding, we have four versions of welfarism. What are the implications of these four approaches for the problem of statistical versus identified lives?

Ex ante utilitarianism, ex post utilitarianism, and the ex post application of an equity-regarding SWF violate PSIV. This is not because they reduce to ranking policies in terms of expected deaths. That is not necessarily true of ex post utilitarianism or the ex post equity-regarding approach, even with the ceteris paribus assumption.[13] Rather, all three approaches are *consequentialist*, in the following sense.

Consequentialism

If, for each state, two policies yield equally good outcomes, the policies are equally good. If, for each state, one policy yields a better outcome than a second, the first policy is better.

Any approach to ranking policies that satisfies Consequentialism, plus an axiom I will call "Death Permutation" (itself an implication of Anonymity), is logically incompatible with PSIV.[14] Using mortality matrices, it is very easy to show this. If Consequentialism and Death Permutation are true, then—in

---

[13] More precisely, with this assumption, that will be true of ex post utilitarianism if the f-function described in the appendix is the identity function or otherwise linear. And it will be true of the ex post equity-regarding approach where the SWF is prioritarian and the f-function is the identity function or otherwise linear. By contrast, Adler, Hammitt, and Treich (2014) show that a concave f-function combined with a utilitarian or prioritarian SWF will be "catastrophe-averse"—rather than focusing on expected deaths.

The rank-weighted SWF is a nonprioritarian but equity-regarding SWF. It can be shown that the ex post approach for this SWF—the expected value of some f-function of the sum of rank-weighed utilities—does not correspond to the minimization of expected deaths even if the f function is the identity function.

[14] Death Permutation says: If individuals are identical in welfare-relevant attributes except whether they live a full life span or die prematurely, and two outcomes have the same number of individuals who die prematurely, the outcomes are equally good.

the case where individuals are identical with respect to nonrisk attributes—a policy that prevents the premature death of one person in a given state is an equal improvement over the status quo as a policy that prevents the premature death of another person in that state—regardless of whether those individuals survive or die prematurely in other states. This forces a conflict with PSIV, as shown in Table 4.3.

TABLE 4.3 } **Consequentialism and PSIV**

Status Quo

	$\pi(s) = .5$	$\pi(s^*) = .5$	Survival Prob.
Able	0	1	.5
Baker	1	0	.5
Charlie	0	0	0

Policy X: *Saving Statistical Victims*

	$\pi(s) = .5$	$\pi(s^*) = .5$	Survival Prob.
Able	1	1	1
Baker	1	1	1
Charlie	0	0	0

Policy Y: *Saving Identified Victim*

	$\pi(s) = .5$	$\pi(s^*) = .5$	Survival Prob.
Able	0	1	.5
Baker	1	0	.5
Charlie	1	1	1

Note: The three tables are mortality matrices, displaying whether each individual lives or dies in a given state. Charlie is an identified victim: in the status quo, he is certain to die prematurely. Able and Baker are statistical victims: each has a status quo chance of .5 of dying prematurely.

Consider the case in which the ceteris paribus assumption holds. PSIV prefers policy *Y* (saving Charlie) to *X* (saving Able and Baker). However, Death Permutation requires indifference between the outcome of *X* and the outcome of *Y* in state *s*, since the same number of individuals die prematurely. Similarly, Death Permutation requires indifference between the outcome of *X* and the outcome of *Y* in state *s**. Thus, Consequentialism requires indifference between policy *X* and policy *Y*—in conflict with PSIV.

By contrast, the ex ante application of an equity-regarding SWF satisfies PSIV. Why? Note first that the ex ante equity-regarding approach satisfies the *ex ante Pigou-Dalton principle*. While the Pigou-Dalton principle mentioned above is a constraint on how SWFs rank outcomes (leaving aside uncertainty), the ex ante Pigou-Dalton principle operates with uncertainty in the picture and says: If the vector of expected utilities associated with a particular policy leaves some individual with less expected utility than a second individual, and we change the policy so that the first individual's expected utility is increased by some amount, the second individual's is reduced by the very same amount, this change shrinks the expected utility gap between the two, and no one else is affected, the new policy is a moral improvement over the original one.

Further, the ex ante Pigou-Dalton principle immediately implies the axiom of Risk Transfer. Finally, Risk Transfer (together with an axiom I will term Risk Permutation, also satisfied by the ex ante application of an SWF) implies PSIV.[15] The proof is provided in the appendix and illustrated in Table 4.4. The risk distribution that results from saving all the statistical victims, and letting the identified victim die, can be converted into the distribution that leaves the statistical victims as is, and saves the identified victim, via a series of risk-gap-diminishing moves.[16]

4. Equity and Uncertainty

Table 4.5 summarizes the analysis to this point, showing how CBA and various SWFs fare with respect to PSIV and other axioms.

If one believes (as does this author) that the best specification of welfarism should be sensitive to equity considerations, and thus embraces some kind of equity-regarding SWF, the problem of identified versus statistical lives reduces to the choice between the last two rows of Table 4.5—the choice between applying an equity-regarding SWF under uncertainty in an "ex post" manner versus doing so in an "ex ante" manner. How should equity-regarding SWFs be applied under conditions of uncertainty? Recapping, the ex post application of an equity-regarding SWF satisfies Consequentialism and thereby violates PSIV, while the ex ante approach satisfies the ex ante Pigou-Dalton principle, thus Risk Transfer, and thereby satisfies PSIV.

It should be noted that the ex ante approach to an equity-regarding SWF under uncertainty might yield, not merely PSIV, but an even more robust priority for identified victims. One kind of equity-regarding SWF is the leximin SWF. Leximin gives absolute priority to improving the position of the worst-off person. Ex ante leximin ranks policies by applying the leximin rule to the vectors of expected utility associated with each policy. Ex ante leximin

---

[15] Risk Permutation says that, if the survival probabilities corresponding to one policy are a permutation of the probabilities corresponding to a second, and the ceteris paribus assumption holds, the policies are equally good.

[16] The reader might wonder how the analysis here is consistent with Bovens and Fleurbaey (2012), an important discussion of ex ante versus ex post approaches to lifesaving. They focus in the main analysis on a two-person population and statistically independent risks; consider various outcome-evaluation functions giving various degrees of extra weight to saving two rather than one individuals; and show that the ex post application of some of these functions actually satisfies ex ante Pigou-Dalton.

Suffice it to say that this last result holds in the case of independent risks. By contrast, PSIV as framed here is a more general axiom, which requires priority for the identified victim regardless of whether the others at risk of dying have independent, correlated, or anticorrelated risks. Table 4.3 shows that no ex post approach—no approach to ranking policies that satisfies Consequentialism—can satisfy PSIV in general. (Note that, in this table, Able and Baker's risks are anticorrelated in the status quo.) Whether a particular SWF, applied ex post, satisfies PSIV in the specific case of independent risks is not a topic I can address here.

TABLE 4.4 } **Risk Transfer and PSIV**

Status Quo	
Able	0
Baker	.95
Charlie	.85
Doug	.7
Eddy	.5

Policy X		Policy I		Policy II		Policy III		Policy Y	
Able	0	Able	.05	Able	.2	Able	.5	Able	1
Baker	1	Baker	.95	Baker	.95	Baker	.95	Baker	.95
Charlie	1	Charlie	1	Charlie	.85	Charlie	.85	Charlie	.85
Doug	1	Doug	1	Doug	1	Doug	.7	Doug	.7
Eddy	1	Eddy	1	Eddy	1	Eddy	1	Eddy	.5

Note: The tables show each individual's survival probability. Able here is the identified victim, while the other individuals are statistical victims. Policy X saves the statistical victims, while Policy Y saves the identified victim. Assume the ceteris paribus premise; then PSIV prefers Y to X. Note that Policy X is converted into Policy I by a transfer of survival probability from Baker to Able; Policy I into Policy II by a transfer from Charlie to Able; and Policy II into Policy III by a transfer from Doug to Able. Thus, the axiom of Risk Transfer requires that Policy III be preferred to Policy II, in turn preferred to Policy I, in turn preferred to Policy X. Finally, Risk Permutation requires indifference between Policy Y and Policy III. By transitivity, Policy Y is preferred to Policy X.

TABLE 4.5 } **A Summary**

	PSIV	Consequentialism	Risk Transfer	Ranking policies in order of expected deaths
Textbook CBA	Yes for one version of textbook CBA; No for the other version	No	No	No
CBA: governmental practice	No	Yes	No	Yes
Ex post utilitarianism	No	Yes	No	Depends on f-function
Ex ante utilitarianism	No	Yes	No	Yes
Ex post equity-regarding SWF	No	Yes	No	Depends on f function and specific SWF
Ex ante equity regarding SWF	Yes	No	Yes	No

Note: This table assumes the ceteris paribus premise (individuals identical in all outcomes except for survival probabilities). Note the implications from Consequentialism to a violation of PSIV; and from Risk Transfer to PSIV. The analysis of Consequentialism assumes that two outcomes with the same number of individuals dying prematurely, differing only in who dies, are equally good; and that an outcome in which fewer individuals die is better than one in which more do. Under the ceteris paribus premise, governmental CBA assigns a cost to each policy equaling the expected number of premature deaths multiplied by a constant VSL; it thus satisfies Consequentialism and ranks policies in the order of expected deaths. On the f-function mentioned here, see note 13 and the appendix.

has two striking implications: (1) With the ceteris paribus assumption held in place, it prefers saving one identified victim to any number of statistical victims, regardless of the reduction in expected deaths from doing the latter (recall that PSIV requires such priority only if the number of expected deaths is reduced by one). (2) If we relax the ceteris paribus assumption, so that the identified victim might have more favorable nonrisk attributes than the statistical victims—but stipulate that premature death is sufficiently bad that the identified victim (if allowed to die) has lower expected utility than any of the statistical victims (if left at risk of death)—ex ante leximin will still require saving the identified victim over any number of statistical victims.

So how should equity be understood? The choice, here, is between fairness in individual expectations and fairness in outcomes. The ex ante approach to applying an equity-regarding SWF is concerned with the distribution of individual expected utilities. This is what the ex ante Pigou-Dalton principle says: An individual with lower expected utility is, in the morally relevant sense, worse off than someone with higher expected utility, and a pure transfer of expected utility that shrinks the gap between them (and affects no one else) is a moral improvement. The ex post approach looks at the distribution of individual utilities in each possible outcome, discounted by the outcome's probability.

I believe the ex ante approach to be problematic, for reasons I have articulated elsewhere (Adler 2012, 506–18). The ex ante Pigou-Dalton principle is inconsistent with Consequentialism. In particular, as illustrated in Table 4.6, ex ante Pigou-Dalton can lead government to favor a policy whose outcome is sure to be worse than the status quo outcome—whatever state of the world results. But this seems irrational.

In sum, welfarists (I believe) should decline to endorse PSIV. They should evaluate policies using the SWF framework (rather than CBA); should adopt an equity-regarding SWF; and should apply that SWF in an ex post manner. This means conforming to Consequentialism and rejecting the priority for identified victims that PSIV requires—even in the ceteris paribus case where the identified and statistical victims are identical with respect to nonrisk attributes, and a fortiori if the reduction in expected deaths from saving the statistical victims exceeds one.

To be sure, proponents of the ex ante application of an equity-regarding SWF can mount a counterattack. They can point out, in particular, that the ex post approach can favor a policy that decreases everyone's expected well-being: it can violate the ex ante Pareto principle. See Table 4.7.

I do not find ex ante Pareto a normatively compelling axiom, but others may. They may prefer to embrace that axiom, together with ex ante Pigou-Dalton, even though this means rejecting Consequentialism (Adler 2012, ch. 7; on welfarist evaluation under uncertainty, see also Fleurbaey 2010; Fleurbaey and Voorhoeve 2013; Mongin and Pivato, forthcoming; Otsuka and Voorhoeve 2009; Parfit 2012).

TABLE 4.6 } **Consequentialism and Ex Ante Pigou Dalton**

	Policy a			Policy b		
	States		Expected Utility	States		Expected Utility
	π(s) = .5	π(s*) = .5		π(s) = .5	π(s*) = .5	
Jim	50	60	55	30	70	50
Sally	50	40	45	70	30	50

Note: The entries in the cells are utility numbers. Note that the Pigou-Dalton principle for ranking outcomes says that the utility vector (30, 70) is worse than the utility vector (50, 50), and that the utility vector (70, 30) is worse than the utility vector (60, 40). Thus (if this principle for ranking outcomes is adopted, as does every equity-regarding SWF), the outcome of policy *a* in each state is better than the outcome of policy *b* in that state. So Consequentialism requires policy *a*, but the ex ante Pigou-Dalton principle requires policy *b*, which equalizes expected utilities relative to policy *a*.

TABLE 4.7 } **A Conflict with Ex Ante Pareto**

	Policy a			Policy b		
	States		Expected Utility	States		Expected Utility
	π(s) = .5	π(s*) = .5		π(s) = .5	π(s*) = .5	
Jim	90	10	50	50 − ε	50 − ε	50 − ε
Sally	10	90	50	50 − ε	50 − ε	50 − ε

Note: As in table 6, the entries in the cells are utility numbers. ε is some positive number. The ex ante Pareto principle prefers policy *a* to policy *b*, since each person's expected utility is greater. However, note that the Pigou-Dalton principle for ranking outcomes says that the utility vector (50, 50) is better than (90, 10) and (10, 90). Thus, an equity-regarding SWF which satisfies that principle as well as an axiom of "continuity" will prefer (50 − ε, 50 − ε) to (90, 10) and (10, 90) if ε is sufficiently small. Given such an SWF, Consequentialism and the ex post approach prefer policy *b*.

I will not attempt, here, to make further headway on the ex post/ex ante debate. Rather, what I have shown is how the problem of statistical versus identified lives is intimately connected to that debate. The welfarist who cares about equity must, further, decide whether the "currency" for fair distribution is expected well-being (the ex ante approach) or final utilities (the ex post approach). And whether she embraces PSIV depends precisely on this.

APPENDIX }

A.1. The Model

Let c be the individual's income during the current period, and $\mathbf{a}$ be all other attributes. $u(c, \mathbf{a})$ is the individual's lifetime utility if she survives the period, and $v(c, \mathbf{a})$ if she dies during the period. Since $\mathbf{a}$ will be identical for all individuals and in all states, as per the ceteris paribus assumption, we can refer to these utility functions as $u(c)$ and $v(c)$. Following the standard model of VSL, we assume that $u(c) > v(c)$, $u'(c) > v'(c) \geq 0$, $u''(c) \leq 0$, $v''(c) \leq 0$. (On this model, see Adler, Hammitt, and Treich 2014, and sources cited therein.)

It is assumed that all individuals have the same preferences. Utility functions $u(.)$ and $v(.)$ are representations of these common preferences. These utility functions will do double duty—they will serve both as the basis for CBA, and as the inputs to SWFs. The SWF approach in general requires interpersonally as well as intrapersonally comparable utilities. Where individuals have common preferences, these unproblematically provide the basis for such comparisons. (One individual is better off than a second iff everyone prefers the first individual's bundle of attributes to the second's.) Interpersonal comparisons become trickier with divergent preferences; such difficulties are ignored here.

A given state s has probability $\pi(s)$. A given governmental policy choice (whether the status quo choice O of inaction, or some alternative choice a) determines, for each individual and state, whether she survives the current period or dies prematurely. Let $l_{i,s}^{O}$ be an indicator variable with value 1 if individual i survives in state s in the status quo, and 0 if she dies prematurely. Similarly, let $l_{i,s}^{a}$ be an indicator variable with value 1 if the individual survives in state s given policy choice a, and 0 if she dies prematurely.

Individual i's survival probability in the status quo, p_i^O, equals $\Sigma_s \pi(s) l_{i,s}^O$. Individual i's expected utility in the status quo, U_i^O, equals $\Sigma_s \pi(s)[l_{i,s}^O u(c) + (1 - l_{i,s}^O) v(c)]$, which in turn just equals $p_i^O u(c) + (1 - p_i^O) v(c)$. Substituting a for O, the same holds true of U_i^a, the individual's expected utility with action a.

A.2. Cost-Benefit Analysis and VSL

In general, CBA ranks policies by summing individuals' equivalent variations or compensating variations. Individual i's *equivalent variation* for a policy a, EV_i^a, is the amount of money such that—were it to be added to her income in every possible status quo outcome—the individual's expected utility in a and O would be the same. Her *compensating variation* for a policy a, CV_i^a, is the amount of money such that—were it to be subtracted from her income in every possible policy outcome—the individual's expected utility in a and O would be the same.

In the simple model at hand, EV_i^a is such that

$$p_i^O u(c + EV_i^a) + (1 - p_i^O) v(c + EV_i^a) = p_i^a u(c) + (1 - p_i^a) v(c).$$

Similarly, CV_i^a is such that

$$p_i^O u(c) + (1-p_i^O)v(c) = p_i^a u(c-CV_i^a) + (1-p_i^a)v(c-CV_i^a).$$

Summing equivalent variations, CBA says policy a is better than the status quo iff $\Sigma_i EV_i^a > 0$. The best way to generalize this rule to the case of multiple alternatives to the status quo is to say that policy a is better than policy b iff $\Sigma_i EV_i^a > \Sigma_i EV_i^b$. Summing compensating variations, CBA follows the same rules except that EV_i is substituted for CV_i.

Let VSL_i denote the marginal rate of substitution between survival probability and wealth in the status quo, that is, $(\partial U_i / \partial p_i)/(\partial U_i / \partial c)$ at the bundle p_i^O, c. Because $U_i^O = p_i^O u(c) + (1-p_i^O)v(c)$, $VSL_i = \dfrac{u(c)-v(c)}{p_i^O u'(c)+(1-p_i^O)v'(c)}$. Since $u'(c) > v'(c)$, it follows that VSL_i decreases with survival probability—the "dead anyway" effect.

For a given policy a, let Δp_i^a denote the reduction in i's fatality risk as compared to the status quo, and ΔU_i^a the change in individual i's expected utility. Then the limit, as Δp_i^a approaches zero, of the ratio $(EV_i^a/\Delta p_i^a)$ is VSL_i. (Observe that this ratio is equal to $\Delta U_i^a/\Delta p_i^a$ divided by $\Delta U_i^a/EV_i^a$.) Moreover, the limit as Δp_i^a approaches zero, of the ratio $(CV_i^a/\Delta p_i^a)$ is also VSL_i. (This follows from the Implicit Function Theorem, Simon and Blume 1994, 339.)

It follows from these observations, plus the fact that CV_i^a and EV_i^a have the same sign as Δp_i^a (positive for a risk reduction, negative for an increase), that if $p_j^O > p_i^O$ and therefore $VSL_j < VSL_i$, (1) the magnitude (absolute value) of individual i's equivalent variation for a policy that changes his fatality risk by Δp will be larger than the magnitude of individual j's equivalent variation for a policy that changes her fatality risk by the same amount, if Δp is sufficiently small; and (2) the magnitude of individual i's compensating variation for a policy that changes his fatality risk by Δp will be larger than the magnitude of individual j's compensating variation for a policy that changes her fatality risk by the same amount, if Δp is sufficiently small. This in turn implies that a policy that reduces i's fatality risk by Δp and increases j's by the same amount will be preferred to the status quo (by both versions of CBA) for all Δp sufficiently small.

A.3. Cost Benefit Analysis, PSIV, and Risk Transfer

Consider the version of CBA that says policy a is better than policy b iff the sum of equivalent variations for a (relative to the status quo) is greater than the sum of equivalent variations for b (relative to the status quo). We now show that this version of CBA satisfies PSIV.

All individuals have income c. Assume that there are M statistical victims in the status quo O, with $M > 1$, numbered 1 through M, such that $p_i^O > 0$ for each such individual, and $\Sigma_{i=1}^M (1 - p_i^O) = 1$. (This last condition is equivalent to saying that saving all the statistical victims reduces the number of expected deaths by 1.) Let k denote the identified victim, such that $p_k^O = 0$. Let X be a policy that saves the statistical victims, that is, $p_i^X = 1$ for each individual i in the group of M, and other individuals' survival probabilities are the same as in the status quo. Let Y be a policy that saves the identified victim, that is, $p_k^Y = 1$, and other individuals' survival probabilities are the same as in the status quo.

Let Δc be the equivalent variation (relative to the status quo) of the identified victim for policy Y, that is, EV_k^Y. Δc is such that $v(c + \Delta c) = u(c)$. Consider some statistical victim i, with baseline probability $p_i^O > 0$ of surviving. To reduce clutter, denote this probability as r, and denote $(1 - r)\Delta c$ as D. Let Δc^+ be the statistical victim's equivalent variation (relative to the status quo) for policy X, that is, EV_i^X. That is, $ru(c + \Delta c^+) + (1 - r)v(c + \Delta c^+) = u(c)$. We now show that $\Delta c^+ < D$.[17]

We will show first that $\Delta c^+ \neq D$. Note that $ru(c + D) = r[u(c + D) - u(c) + u(c)]$. Because $u' > v'$ at all income levels, $u(c + D) - u(c) > v(c + D) - v(c)$, and thus $r[u(c + D) - u(c) + u(c)] > r[v(c + D) - v(c) + u(c)]$. Adding $(1 - r)v(c + D)$ to both sides, and simplifying, we have

$$ru(c+D)+(1-r)v(c+D) > v(c+D)+r[u(c)-v(c)] \qquad (1)$$

Note, now, that $c + D = rc + (1 - r)(c + \Delta c)$. Because $v'' \leq 0$, $v(rc + (1 - r)(c + \Delta c)) \geq rv(c) + (1 - r) v(c + \Delta c) = rv(c) + (1 - r) u(c)$. Thus

$$v(c+D) \geq rv(c)+(1-r)u(c). \qquad (2)$$

Putting (1) and (2) together, it follows that $r(u(c + D)) + (1 - r)v(c + D) > u(c)$. This shows that $\Delta c^+ \neq D$. Moreover, because $v' \geq 0$ and $u' > 0$, it cannot be the case that $\Delta c^+ > D$.

The sum of equivalent variations for Y is just Δc. The sum of equivalent variations for X is $\Sigma_{i=1}^M EV_i^X$. We have just demonstrated that $EV_i^X < (1 - p_i^O) \Delta c$. Thus $\Sigma_{i=1}^M EV_i^X < \Sigma_{i=1}^M (1 - p_i^O) \Delta c = \Delta c$.

However, this version of CBA does not satisfy the axiom of Risk Transfer. The key difficulty is this. Individual j (the person with the lower fatality risk in

---

[17] Δc will only be a finite number if $v' > 0$, which means either that the individual who dies in the current period will be able to use that income during the period, or that it has some "bequest value" to him. Alternatively, if Δc is infinite—and, in addition, $\Delta c+$ is finite for every statistical victim—CBA will view the identified victim's death as incompensable and, in that way, will give priority to saving her.

policy a, as per the axiom) may have a larger equivalent variation for policy a than individual i. (This will not happen of course if policy a is just the status quo, but it can happen otherwise.) But under the simple model here, willingness to pay for risk reduction is increasing with income—so it is possible that the change in EV_j^a necessary to make j indifferent between the status quo and policy b is greater than the change in EV_i^a.

For a concrete example of how this version of CBA violates Risk Transfer, let $v(c) = \ln c$ and $u(c) = 2v(c)$, with $c > 1$. Assume that all individuals have income 100, and that in the status quo both individuals i and j have survival probability .3. Let policy a be such their survival probabilities are, respectively, .1 and .9; while policy b is such that their survival probabilities are .4 and .6. Everyone else has the same survival probabilities in policy a and b. Then Risk Transfer prefers policy b. However, it can be verified that individual i and j have equivalent variations for policy a of, respectively, −51 and 738; while their equivalent variations for policy b are 43 and 189. Thus, the sum of equivalent variations prefers policy a.

For a showing that this version of CBA will satisfy Risk Transfer in the special case where policy a is the status quo, see Adler, Hammitt, and Treich 2014.

What about CBA in the version that ranks policies by summing compensating variations relative to the status quo? This version does not satisfy Risk Transfer, even in the special case where a is the status quo. See Adler, Hammitt, and Treich 2014. Nor does it satisfy PSIV. For a counterexample, again let $v(c) = \ln c$ and $u(c) = 2v(c)$, with $c > 1$. Assume that $c = 100$ and that in the status quo there are two statistical victims each with a probability of .5 of dying, and one identified victim. Then it can be verified that the identified victim's compensating variation for being saved is 90, while each of the statistical victim's compensating variations is 68.38, twice which exceeds 90.

A.4. Risk Transfer plus Risk Permutation Implies PSIV

As above, assume that there are M statistical victims in the status quo O, with $M > 1$, numbered 1 through M, such that $p_i^O > 0$ for each such individual, and $\sum_{i=1}^{M}(1 - p_i^O) = 1$. Let k denote the identified victim, such that $p_k^O = 0$. X and Y are as above, with X saving the statistical victims and Y the identified victim, and other individuals having the same survival probabilities as in the status quo

Consider a series of M policies $a(0), a(1), a(2), \ldots, a(m), \ldots, a(M)$, constructed as follows: (1) policy $a(0) = X$. (2) Given $m > 0$, policy $a(m)$ is such that $p_i^{a(m)} = p_i^O$ for $i \leq m$, and $p_i^{a(m)} = 1$ for $i > m$, $i \leq M$; and for individual k, her survival probability in $a(m)$, $p_k^{a(m)}$, equals $\sum_{i=1}^{m}(1 - p_i^O)$. (Individuals other than the statistical and identical victims have the same survival probabilities as in the status quo.) Note that $a(M) = Y$.

By Risk Transfer, policy $a(m)$ is preferred to policy $a(m-1)$ for $m = 1$ to $M - 1$. Why? Note that the survival probability of individual k with policy $a(m-1)$ is $\Sigma_{i=1}^{m-1}(1-p_i^O)$, while the survival probability of individual m is 1. With policy $a(m)$, individual k's survival probability is $\Sigma_{i=1}^{m}(1-p_i^O)$ and individual m's survival probability is p_m^O—so that k's survival probability has increased by $(1-p_m^O)$, while individual m's survival probability has decreased by the same amount. Finally, because $p_k^{a(m)} < 1$, the gap between the two survival probabilities has shrunk.

Finally, note that the survival probabilities in $a(M-1)$ are a permutation of the survival probabilities in $a(M) = Y$, so that by Risk Permutation, $a(M-1)$ is as good as $a(M)$. Because $a(m)$ is better than $a(m-1)$ for $m = 1$ to $M-1$, and $a(M) = Y$ is equally good as $a(M-1)$, it follows by transitivity that Y is better than $a(0) = X$.

A.5. Social Welfare Functions and Consequentialism

Returning from our simple model to a more general setup, let $x^{a,s}$ be the outcome of policy a in state s. Let $u_i(x^{a,s})$ be the utility of individual i in that outcome. Let U_i^a be individual i's expected utility with policy a, that is, $\Sigma_s \pi(s) u_i(x^{a,s})$. Then ex ante utilitarianism assigns a given policy a the number $\Sigma_i U_i^a$, and ranks policies according to these numbers. Ex post utilitarianism assigns a given policy a the number $\Sigma_s \pi(s) f(\Sigma_i u_i(x^{a,s}))$, with f an increasing function. Note that ex ante utilitarianism is equivalent to ex post utilitarianism if f is the identity function.

An equity-regarding SWF may (but need not) be representable by a function w, such that the SWF weakly prefers one utility vector $(u_1, \ldots, u_i, \ldots, u_N)$ to another $(u_1^*, \ldots, u_i^*, \ldots, u_N^*)$ iff $w(u_1, \ldots, u_i, \ldots, u_N) \geq w(u_1^*, \ldots, u_i^*, \ldots, u_N^*)$. The leximin SWF is an example of an equity-regarding SWF that is not thus representable, as is the prioritarian SWF with a lexical threshold.

The ex ante approach to applying a given equity-regarding SWF is straightforward: it takes the rule for ranking utility vectors just mentioned, and applies it to the vectors of expected utilities associated with each policy. Policy a is at least as good as policy b just in case $(U_1^a, \ldots, U_N^a)$ is weakly preferred by the rule to $(U_1^b, \ldots, U_N^b)$.

As for the ex post approach: Let $\mathbf{U}(x)$ be the vector of utility numbers associated with outcome x. If the equity-regarding SWF is representable by a function w, then the ex post equity-regarding approach assigns a given policy a the number $\Sigma_s \pi(s) f(w(\mathbf{U}(x^{a,s})))$, with f an increasing function.

It is clear from these definitions that ex post utilitarianism (hence ex ante utilitarianism, equivalent to one version thereof) and the ex post equity-regarding approach (with the SWF representable by w) satisfy Consequentialism. Outcomes are "better" or "equally good" according to the underlying SWF. Thus, in the case of ex post utilitarianism, two outcomes are equally good if they have the same sum of utilities, and one outcome is better if it has a greater sum of utilities. In the case of ex post equity-regard, two outcomes are equally good if they have the same w-value, and one is better if it has a greater w-value.

If the SWF is not representable by a w function, then the "ex post" approach means any rule for ranking policies that satisfies Consequentialism (given the ranking of outcomes generated by that SWF). See Fleurbaey 2010, describing ex post approaches to applying the leximin SWF.

References

Adler, M. D. 2004. "Fear Assessment: Cost-Benefit Analysis and the Pricing of Fear and Anxiety." *Chicago-Kent Law Review* 79: 977–1053.
Adler, M. D. 2012. *Well-Being and Fair Distribution: Beyond Cost-Benefit Analysis*. New York: Oxford University Press.
Adler, M. D. 2013. "Happiness Surveys and Public Policy: What's the Use?" *Duke Law Journal* 62: 1509–601.
Adler, M. D., and E. A. Posner. 2006. *New Foundations of Cost-Benefit Analysis*. Cambridge, MA: Harvard University Press.
Adler, M. D., J. K. Hammitt, and N. Treich. 2014. "The Social Value of Mortality Risk Reduction: VSL versus the Social Welfare Function Approach." *Journal of Health Economics* 35: 82–93.
Bossert, W., and J. A. Weymark. 2004. "Utility in Social Choice." In *Handbook of Utility Theory*, vol. 2, *Extensions*, edited by S. Barberà et al., 1099–177. Boston: Kluwer.
Bovens, L., and M. Fleurbaey. 2012. "Evaluating Life or Death Prospects." *Economics and Philosophy* 28: 217–49.
Fleurbaey, M. 2010. "Assessing Risky Social Situations." *Journal of Political Economy* 118: 649–80.
Fleurbaey, M., and A. Voorhoeve. 2013. "Decide as You Would with Full Information! An Argument against Ex Ante Pareto." In *Inequalities in Health: Concepts, Measures, and Ethics*, edited by N. Eyal, S. A. Hurst, Ole F. Norheim, and Dan Wikler, 113–28. Oxford: Oxford University Press.
Mongin, P., and M. Pivato. Forthcoming. "Social Preference and Social Welfare under Risk and Uncertainty." In *Oxford Handbook of Well-Being and Public Policy*, edited by M. D. Adler and M. Fleurbaey. New York: Oxford University Press.
Otsuka, M., and A. Voorhoeve. 2009. "Why It Matters That Some Are Worse Off Than Others: An Argument against the Priority View." *Philosophy and Public Affairs* 37: 171–99.
Parfit, D. 2012. "Another Defence of the Priority View." *Utilitas* 24: 399–440.

Robinson, L. 2007. "How U.S. Government Agencies Value Mortality Risk Reductions," *Review of Environmental Economics and Policy* 1: 283–99.

Simon, C. P, and L. Blume. 1994. *Mathematics for Economists*. New York: Norton.

5 }

Risking Life and Limb
HOW TO DISCOUNT HARMS BY THEIR IMPROBABILITY
Michael Otsuka

1.

Suppose that a comet carrying a pathogen has landed in a cornfield in the American Midwest. The government soon comes to realize that it is faced with the following three options:

Do Nothing: Doing nothing, in which case it is known that this pathogen would wipe out 100,000 people who live within a 500-mile radius of this cornfield, while sparing everyone outside of this radius.

Sacrifice Known Limb: Taking steps that would be effective in preventing this plague, but at the foreseen and unintended cost of one person's limb. It is known in advance who this person would be: a particular individual named Bob who lives in Boca Raton, Florida.

Sacrifice Unknown Life (dust): Taking steps that would be equally effective in preventing this plague, but at the foreseen and unintended cost of another person's life. It is not known by anyone in advance who this person would be. All that is known is that he would be someone who resides in California (population circa 40 million). Moreover, let us stipulate that his death would be causally necessitated by the measures taken to combat the pathogen, and the death of anyone else would be causally impossible. We might imagine that these measures would result in the release of a cloud of rare and exotic particles of dust that would descend on California, leaving everyone completely unaffected except for one person whose unique genetic constitution would doom him to a fatal adverse reaction to these particles. In other words, it is objectively determined, but not known by anyone, which person would die. When we consider their epistemic risks—that is, those risks we are justified in believing to be the case, given the evidence available to us—each Californian would be exposed to an equal and very small 1 in 40 million chance of being killed.[1]

One could not justify subjecting each Californian to this slight risk of death, or subjecting Bob in Boca Raton to the certainty of harm short of death, on grounds that this would be better for them than doing nothing. Leaving aside any self-regarding interest people in Florida or California might have in the fate of Midwesterners, elimination of the plague is not in their interests, given that they all lie outside of the 500-mile radius of the comet's impact and hence are unthreatened by the pathogen.[2] It is nevertheless clear that the government must do something. So many lives would be lost if the government did nothing, and these lives could be saved at such a relatively small cost to others, that the case against doing nothing is overwhelming. So we should remove *Do Nothing* from the agenda.

What about the remaining two options: *Sacrifice Known Limb* and *Sacrifice Unknown Life (dust)*, where *Sacrifice Known Limb* would deprive Bob in Boca Raton of a limb, and *Sacrifice Unknown Life (dust)* would kill our unknown Californian? Intuitively, it seems that we should sacrifice Bob's limb rather than a Californian's life. But suppose that we adopt a familiar method of discounting harms by their known improbability, whereby we simply multiply the magnitude of a harm someone would suffer by the known probability of his suffering it. We often discount harms in such fashion, in order to try to justify the imposition of risks on those who do not benefit from the risky activity. This, for example, is how one might try to justify some risks arising from flights over isolated aboriginal islanders in the Andaman Sea: although these flights expose each islander to a risk of being killed by a malfunctioning

---

[1] This example was inspired by an example of Sophia Reibetanz's (1998, 302). In her example, if you do nothing, one of a group of 100 peasants is certain to lose a limb to a land mine while tilling the soil, though nobody knows in advance which peasant this will be. You can deactivate this land mine, but at the inevitable cost of your coming down with pneumonia, which is stipulated to be one-tenth as bad as losing a limb. Reibetanz's example raises questions regarding the nature and extent of the duties that private individuals have to come to the assistance of strangers, plus related questions regarding the countervailing agent-relative permission they might have to give greater weight to their own interests rather than those of strangers. My example shifts the focus from private duties of beneficence to public obligations regarding the distribution of risks and harms. In so doing, it also renders questions regarding agent-relative prerogatives irrelevant, because we are no longer asking to what lengths a private individual must go in order to assist others. Rather, we are asking what sorts of duties public officials have when it comes to the distribution of harm or risks of harms among its citizens.

[2] It is a vexing question whether and, if so, when a risky course of action can be justified on the grounds that it is in the expected self-interest of individuals to be exposed to such risks, given the benefits to which such exposure gives rise. I shall sidestep this question by considering only cases of risk-imposition that are not in the expected interest of those exposed to the risks. Throughout this chapter, I shall also limit myself to a consideration of harms and risks of harm that are merely foreseen and shall therefore set to one side the special case in which the harmful or risky use of some is intended as a means to a greater good.

falling plane, the probability is sufficiently miniscule for each that we feel that it is justifiable to subject him to such a risk.[3] If we apply this type of discounting to the two options under consideration, it would follow that none of the residents of California would have a complaint that is as great as the complaint of Bob in Boca Raton. That is because each Californian's complaint against dying as the result of *Sacrifice Unknown Life (dust)* would be sharply discounted by the 1 in 40 million chance that he would die prematurely. Premature death is undoubtedly worse than losing a limb. But it is not 40 million times worse. It would, after all, be rational for a person to expose himself to far higher than a 1 in 40 million risk of losing his life in order to save a limb that he would otherwise be certain to lose.

Even if one acknowledges that each Californian's probability-discounted complaint against losing a life is much smaller than Bob's undiscounted complaint against losing a limb, one might argue that the government should nevertheless choose *Sacrifice Known Limb* over *Sacrifice Unknown Life (dust)* for the following reason: even though each Californian's complaint is very small because heavily discounted, when these 40 million complaints are gathered together and aggregated, they are collectively great enough to outweigh the undiscounted complaint of Bob in Boca Raton against losing his limb. I would resist this line of argument. Such aggregation invokes the wrong rationale here. As I shall explain in the next two paragraphs, it is either an appeal to morally trivial considerations or else superfluous.

Once it has been so heavily discounted, each Californian's complaint against death becomes something fairly trivial: the complaint against a subjection to a miniscule increase in one's risk of premature death that is no greater than various risks of premature death we accept as a matter of course in exchange for small conveniences. Such complaints might be regarded as so trivial as to be morally irrelevant when compared with serious complaints (see Kamm 1993, chs. 8–9). We would not, for example, want to allow the mere annoyance of millions over missing 15 minutes of a World Cup match to outweigh the claim of one person in the television transmitter room to be spared the suffering of "extremely painful electrical shocks."[4] Moreover, a person might well prefer a very slight, 1 in 40 million, increase in his odds of premature death to the certainty of 15 minutes of annoyance and frustration from an interrupted World Cup broadcast. Suppose, for example, that our World Cup viewers each knew that shouting at his blank television screen would cause his set to resume broadcasting even though he also knew that such shouting would very, very slightly increased his existing risk of a fatal heart attack by that extra increment, as it well might. I doubt that this health warning would deter people

---

[3] Here I set to one side the more indirect, and probably far more serious, risks arising from climate change that air travel imposes on these islanders.
[4] This memorable example is T. M. Scanlon's (1998, 235).

from shouting at their televisions, and such shouting might even be rational under the circumstances.

There is, to be sure, the following important difference between Scanlon's World Cup case and my own example of Californians placed at risk in *Sacrifice Unknown Life (dust)*. In my case of Californians at risk, the trivially low risks of death shared by millions together constitute something very far from trivial: the certainty of a death. By contrast, millions of viewers' experiencing annoyance and frustration over an interrupted World Cup match do not together constitute any serious harm to anyone. But this difference between Scanlon's World Cup case and my case of Californians at risk reveals that it is superfluous to aggregate the individually minor complaints of the many Californians. Rather, it is sufficient merely to appeal to the strength of the nondiscounted complaint of the one Californian who would die in order to justify *Sacrifice Known Limb* over *Sacrifice Unknown Life (dust)*. If the government opts for *Sacrifice Unknown Life (dust)*, one particular Californian with the unique genetic constitution is certain to die, and this person would have an objective 100% chance of dying.[5] He shares the same objective 100% chance of being harmed under *Sacrifice Unknown Life (dust)* that Bob in Boca Raton has of being harmed under *Sacrifice Known Limb*. Given that they each share an objective certainty of being harmed under the respective courses of action, shouldn't we simply compare the magnitude of the two harms—premature death for the Californian versus the loss of a limb for Bob in Boca Raton—without discounting this particular Californian's harm by its epistemic improbability?

We should pause to ask ourselves why it is that our unknown Californian with the unique genetic constitution who is fated to die nevertheless shares the same epistemic and very low 1 in 40 million risk of dying as every other Californian. The answer to this question is that it is simply on account of our inability to pick this unfortunate individual out of a crowd of 40 million Californians. This shared low epistemic probability of dying seems morally irrelevant, given the apparent unreality of these merely epistemic risks that he shares with every other Californian. Our inability due to ignorance to pick him out of a

---

[5] Throughout this chapter, what I shall mean by "objective probability" is "frequencies relative to classes of events and persons . . . that [in fact] share all the [same] causally relevant features—not merely the features about which good statistical data is actually available." Here I adopt Matthew Adler's frequentist definition of "physical probability" (Adler 2003, 1352). He contrasts such probability with what he calls "statistical probability," which is defined as frequencies relative to classes of events and persons about which statistical data is actually available (Adler 2003, 1348–53). I shall call this "epistemic" rather than "statistical" probability. Some might object to my labelling different subsets of frequentist probabilities "objective" and "epistemic" on grounds that, for frequentists, all probabilities count as objective, in contrast to rival Bayesians, who regard all probabilities as epistemic. There seems a clear sense, however, in which what Adler calls "physical probability" is objective, since it is just a matter of the way the world is. There is also a clear sense in which what he labels statistical probability is epistemic, since it is a matter of what we can know, given the evidence available to us.

large crowd, in contrast with our ability to single out the identity of Bob in Boca Raton, should not make such a big difference to the strength of their claims against being harmed. It seems right that we assign this unknown Californian a nondiscounted 100% complaint against death just as we assign Bob in Boca Raton a nondiscounted 100% complaint against losing a limb. Here it appears that we should assign our unknown Californian a complaint that tracks his 100% *objective* risk of death rather than one that tracks his *merely epistemic* 1 in 40 million risk of death. Once we do so, our choice boils down to the following: imposing loss of limb on one person under *Sacrifice Known Limb* or imposing loss of life on another person under *Sacrifice Unknown Life (dust)*. Once things have been appropriately framed in this manner, it becomes clear that we should spare a life rather than a limb and therefore that we should choose *Sacrifice Known Limb*.

2.

In arguing that we should not discount our unknown Californian's complaint by its epistemic improbability, I have appealed to the apparent greater significance of objective rather than epistemic improbabilities when the two differ. But what should we say about a scenario in which epistemic and objective probabilities fail to come apart in the manner of the scenario we have been considering to this point? Let us now suppose that, instead of the option of *Sacrifice Unknown Life (dust)*, we have the option of subjecting Californians to a different sort of risk, which I shall call *Sacrifice Unknown Life (wheel)*. Here it is certain that precisely one Californian would die if you exposed them to this risk, yet he and everyone else would have an objective, and not merely an epistemic, 1 in 40 million chance of dying. We can stipulate that *Sacrifice Unknown Life (wheel)* would have the following foreseen but unintended consequence: each person would be exposed to a risk that, insofar as its causal nature is concerned, is equivalent to the following scenario that I invite you to imagine: as the result of natural processes, a large ball would receive a hard but indeterministic push that would cause it to spin around and around a very large roulette wheel in the sky that contains 40 million slots. Each slot is connected to a chute that leads to a unique Californian. The ball would eventually travel down one of these 40 million chutes, thereby killing the person to which it leads. Here each Californian would have an objective as well as an epistemic 1 in 40 million chance of dying. It is not deterministically fated in advance that any particular Californian would die. It is, however, known in advance that precisely one Californian would die.

Unlike the option of *Sacrifice Unknown Life (dust)*, under the option of *Sacrifice Unknown Life (wheel)* it is not simply due to our ignorance as to which one of the 40 million Californians would be killed that we assign each of them a 1 in 40 million chance of premature death. Rather, this reflects a genuine objective risk that each of them shares to precisely the same degree of being hit by a big roulette ball from the sky. Each Californian is placed at risk by being underneath this roulette wheel in the sky. By contrast, no Californian is placed at any genuine risk simply by being part of the crowd into which the one man with the unique genetic constitution has been lost. The 1 in 40 million odds of dying a premature death that we assign to each under *Sacrifice Unknown Life (dust)* reflects just our lack of information about the way the world really is rather than any exposure to dangers that the world presents to each.

It might be sensible to conclude, on the basis of these differences, that we possess good reason in *Sacrifice Unknown Life (wheel)*, and that good reason is lacking in *Sacrifice Unknown Life (dust)*, to take seriously the 1 in 40 million risk that each Californian would have of suffering premature death. This is not enough, however, to establish that complaints against *Sacrifice Unknown Life (wheel)* should track nothing other than this genuine risk: that is, that we should sharply discount every Californian's complaint by the very low probability that he in particular would suffer it in this case. Although I have offered grounds to assign each Californian in *Sacrifice Unknown Life (wheel)* a complaint against premature death that is discounted by its 1 in 40 million chance of coming about in his case, I have not also offered any reason to exclude the following further and much more significant complaint: that of the one Californian who would be killed by the falling roulette ball. Perhaps he has a nondiscounted complaint against being killed.

If we take account of his complaint against being killed, while also taking account of every Californian's complaint against being subjected to an objective risk of being killed, might we be accused of double-counting? I do not think this accusation has force. This is because it is morally objectionable both to be killed and to be subjected to an objective risk of being killed that does not result in any tangible physical harm. You have a complaint, for example, against having Russian roulette played on you even if this does not result in your being killed.[6] If, moreover, you are killed as the result of having Russian roulette played on you, then you have a distinct and far more serious complaint.

To be sure, the complaint of the Californian who would be killed under *Sacrifice Unknown Life (wheel)* differs, in the following respect, from the complaint of the person who would be killed under *Sacrifice Unknown Life (dust)*: *Sacrifice Unknown Life (dust)* would kill someone and subject that person to an objective 100% chance of being killed, whereas *Sacrifice*

---

[6] This complaint is more than a matter of the anxiety you might suffer as the result of having risks imposed on you. You would have a serious complaint against the person who played Russian roulette on you even if he did so while you were asleep.

Unknown Life (wheel) would kill someone while subjecting that person (along with every other Californian) to a much lower 1 in 40 million objective chance of being killed. In this respect, *Sacrifice Unknown Life (dust)* is more analogous than *Sacrifice Unknown Life (wheel)* to *Sacrifice Known Limb*: like the uniquely genetically constituted man in *Sacrifice Unknown Life (dust)*, Bob in Boca Raton would both be harmed and subjected to a 100% objective chance of being harmed.

The fact that Bob would be subjected to a 100% objective chance of being harmed, whereas the objective risks of harm would be spread widely, thinly, and equally across all Californians in *Sacrifice Unknown Life (wheel)*, provides a respect in which Bob would have a complaint that nobody would have in *Sacrifice Unknown Life (wheel)*: namely, that he, but no Californian, would bear a very high objective risk of incurring serious harm. I do not think, however, that such a complaint of high objective risk should count for all that much in and of itself. It is, for example, not all that much worse for you to be killed after being shot point blank from the barrel of a gun that was sure to fire a bullet than it is to be killed as the result of having Russian roulette played on you, where the objective risk was only one in six.

I grant that it would be better, because a more egalitarian spreading of burdens, if, other things equal, objective risks were spread equally rather than unequally. If, for example, we were faced with a choice between *Sacrifice Unknown Life (wheel)* and *Sacrifice Unknown Life (dust)*, then we would have reason to choose the former insofar as the burden of the objective risks that people would bear would be more evenly and therefore equally spread than under the latter. But the fact that objective risks would be equally spread should not count for that much. For suppose that under *Sacrifice Unknown Life (dust)* the one who would be harmed would suffer quadriplegia rather than death. Faced with a choice between, on the one hand, *Sacrifice Unknown Life (wheel)*, which is certain to kill someone, and, on the other hand, this variant of *Sacrifice Unknown Life (dust)*, which is certain to render one person a quadriplegic, it would not be right to choose the former over the latter even though the genuine risks of serious harm are more equally spread under *Sacrifice Unknown Life (wheel)* than under this variant of *Sacrifice Unknown Life (dust)*. Rather, we should minimize tangible harms by choosing to spare one person from death rather than one person from quadriplegia.[7]

---

[7] It is also worth noting that the equal spreading, as opposed to an unequal concentration, of objective risks might lead to a greater incidence of fear and anxiety, assuming that people are aware of the risks they face. Even though, for example, objective risks are spread more equally when each of two people is subjected to a known, objective 50% chance of death than when one is exposed to a known, objective 100% of death and the other to a known, objective zero chance of death, there is arguably a greater sum total of fear and anxiety in the former case as compared with the latter. I owe this point to Harry Adamson.

The following is the most morally significant fact about *Sacrifice Unknown Life (wheel)*: even though anyone who would end up being killed by the falling roulette ball had a very low 1 in 40 million objective probability of being killed, there is, under this course of action, an objective 100% certainty that someone—and, moreover, that precisely one person—would be killed by the falling roulette ball. I would like to propose that what explains why we should not discount the complaint against being killed of our unknown Californian under *Sacrifice Unknown Life (wheel)* is the fact that there is, under *Sacrifice Unknown Life (wheel)*, as under *Sacrifice Unknown Life (dust)*, an objective 100% certainty that *someone* would be killed. Moreover, since Bob would have less of a complaint against the sacrifice of his arm in *Sacrifice Known Limb* than our unknown Californian who is certain to be killed would have against the sacrifice of his life in *Sacrifice Unknown Life (wheel)*, the government ought to do that which results in the loss of Bob's arm rather than the loss of the Californian's life.

3.

There is a challenge to this line of reasoning that I shall now present and then surmount. This challenge has to do with the metaphysics of open counterfactuals. It can be formulated as follows. Suppose that the government chooses *Sacrifice Known Limb*. This gives rise to a serious complaint on the part of Bob. If, however, the government had done otherwise by opting for *Sacrifice Unknown Life (wheel)*, then no particular flesh-and-blood Californian would have had a complaint. This is because, for each and every one of the 40 million actual flesh-and-blood Californians, picked out by Social Security number, none of the following counterfactuals is true: "Had the government opted for *Sacrifice Unknown Life (wheel)*, the Californian who would have been killed would have been the person with Social Security number x." None of the 40 million counterfactual conditionals that posits a particular Californian who would have been killed is true because it is never made determinate who this person would be. No such counterfactual is true for the same reason that neither of the following two counterfactuals is true: (1) "Had I indeterministically tossed a coin just now, it would have landed heads," and (2) "Had I indeterministically tossed a coin just now, it would have landed tails." None of these counterfactuals is true for the following reason: there is no way the world ever goes to make actual any one of the equally likely scenarios involving roulette balls or coin landings.[8]

---

[8] For more on the metaphysics of open counterfactuals, and for discussion of their normative significance, see Hare (2012).

We need to draw a distinction between such open counterfactuals regarding ways the world *never goes* from the following analogous future contingents regarding ways the world has not yet but *will go*. If I will, in fact, reach into my pocket and indeterministically toss a coin between now and the moment you finish reading this paragraph, there is a particular way in which it will land, though this is not yet settled. Similarly, if the government will, in fact, opt for *Sacrifice Unknown Life (wheel)*, there is a particular flesh-and-blood Californian who will be killed, though this is not yet settled. If, however, I will not reach into my pocket and toss a coin before you finish reading this paragraph, then there is nothing ever to settle the matter how the coin would land, were I, contrary to fact, to reach into my pocket and toss it before then. Similarly, if the government opts for the sacrifice of Bob's arm rather than the sacrifice of a Californian's life, then there is nothing ever to settle the matter which particular Californian would have been killed had the government chosen otherwise.

There are certain things that are settled regarding the person who would have been killed by a falling roulette ball. It is settled, for example, that the person would have been a Californian. But the Californian who would have been killed lacks a particular Social Security number, gender, town of origin, precise date of birth, and so forth. The person would have had a Social Security number, would have been either a man or a woman, and so forth, but there is no fact of the matter which in particular. In this respect, the person is akin to a fictional character rather than an actual flesh-and-blood human being like you or me or each of the 40 million actual Californians. For each of us, there is a fact of the matter whether we have an even or an odd number of hair follicles at any given point in time. The fictional character Hamlet also has either an even or an odd number of hair follicles at any given point in time, but there is never any fact of the matter whether the number is ever odd or even in Hamlet's case.

Our abstract Californian with the complaint against being killed by the roulette ball is even less determinate than a fictional character such as Hamlet, since, unlike Hamlet, he or she lacks a particular determinate gender, a particular determinate disposition toward self-pity and indecision, and so on. One might wonder how much moral standing the complaint of such an abstract entity could have. There is a memorable line that Woody Allen gives the Mia Farrow character in *The Purple Rose of Cairo*: "I just met the most wonderful man.... He's fictional, but you can't have everything!" It is certainly not everything. But is it even enough? The complaint of the "one Californian" who would die that moves the government to sacrifice Bob's arm seems to be the phantom complaint of a purely abstract entity who is not identical to any one of the 40 million actual Californians. Is the complaint of our abstract Californian against losing his life really enough to override actual flesh-and-blood Bob's complaint against losing his own flesh and blood—that is, his arm?

One might question whether the complaints of such abstract entities, who are other than any actual persons, have moral force. We do not, for example, give moral weight to claims of merely possible persons to be brought in to existence and experience fulfilling lives. (Parents need not be moved to conceive another, and another, etc., child, by the complaints of such possible persons.) Unlike in the case of a merely possible person who is not brought into existence, where no actual person suffers any harm from the parents' decision not to conceive, an actual flesh-and-blood person would have suffered harm if the roulette ball had been unleashed. But since that actual person appears not to be identical to any one of the 40 million Californians, one might wonder whether such an abstraction has moral standing to complain. For any one of the 40 million actual flesh-and-blood Californians, it appears, moreover, that his or her complaint is nothing stronger than that he or she might, but with only a 1 in 40 million chance, have died if you had opted for *Sacrifice Unknown Life (wheel)*. Each actual Californian's complaint therefore seems less serious than Bob's complaint.

So how, then, can we justify the conviction that the government ought to sacrifice Bob's arm rather than one Californian's life? I believe that the answer to this question is that the complaint of the one Californian who would lose his life is not the complaint of an indeterminate person along the lines of a fictional character. We should not conceive of this person as along the lines of Benjamin Braddock, the fictional character played by Dustin Hoffman in the film version of *The Graduate*, who is a Californian, presumably alive today, yet nonidentical to any of the 40 million actual Californians. Rather the indeterminacy of the person is simply the lack of determinacy as to which of the 40 million equally likely scenarios would have been the upshot, where each scenario involves the killing of an actual flesh-and-blood Californian with a particular Social Security number, a specific, fully filled-in life history, and so on. In spite of this indeterminacy, we know that if we had opted for *Sacrifice Unknown Life (wheel)*, there certainly would have been an actual flesh-and-blood person who would have been killed. It is that objective 100% chance that one such scenario would eventuate, involving the killing of a particular actual flesh-and-blood Californian, that grounds the claim that the complaint of the person who would be killed by the falling roulette ball should not be discounted.

4.

Let us now consider another option, which I shall call *Sacrifice Unknown Number of Lives (guns)*. Here the averting of the plague would have the following unintended side-effect: each Californian would be subjected to an objective 1 in 40 million risk of premature death. Moreover, insofar as the causal nature of this risk is concerned, this course of action is equivalent to the following scenario that I invite you to imagine: there are 40 million guns, each of whose barrels is pointed at a unique Californian. Each gun contains one bullet, which resides in one of its 40 million chambers. The cylinder would be spun at an extremely high velocity and the trigger would eventually be pulled. The velocity of the spin and the timing of the pulling of the trigger are set by indeterministic natural processes. As was true of *Sacrifice Unknown Life (wheel)*, in *Sacrifice Unknown Number of Lives (guns)* each Californian would have an objective and not just an epistemic 1 in 40 million chance of dying prematurely. Both scenarios differ, therefore, from *Sacrifice Unknown Life (dust)*, in which everyone would, objectively speaking, either be certain to die prematurely or certain to be spared this fate, and their 1 in 40 million chances of dying are merely epistemic. *Sacrifice Unknown Number of Lives (guns)* differs, however, from both *Sacrifice Unknown Life (dust)* and *Sacrifice Unknown Life (wheel)* in the following respect: it would be fated, under both *Sacrifice Unknown Life (dust)* and *Sacrifice Unknown Life (wheel)*, that precisely one individual would die. This would not be so-fated under *Sacrifice Unknown Number of Lives (guns)*. Rather, as each person's objective chances would be independent of every other person's chances in this scenario, there would be no guarantee that one person would die. There is a decent chance that an empty chamber would align with the barrel of the gun on each occasion and therefore that nobody would die.[9] There is also some chance that more than one would die—in fact, a vanishingly small chance that every single Californian would die.

Sophia Reibetanz has fixed on the moral significance of the presence versus the absence of certainty that anyone would be harmed as the result of our acting on a given principle regarding the imposition of risks. She writes:

> [W]e must reject the proposal that whenever we cannot identify in advance those who will be affected by acceptance of a principle, we should assign each individual a complaint based upon his expected effects. Rather, we should follow this suggestion: as long as we know that acceptance of a principle will affect someone in a certain way, we should assign that person a complaint that is based upon the full magnitude of the harm or benefit, even if we cannot identify the person in advance. It is only if we do not know whether acceptance of a principle will affect anyone in a certain way that we should allocate each individual a complaint based upon his expected harms and benefits under that principle. (Reibetanz 1998, 304)

Reibetanz also maintains that "[o]f course, when we do not know whether anyone will be affected in a certain way by acceptance of some principle,

---

[9] This chance is 1 in e—or about 37%.

then the best we can do is to calculate the complaint of each person on the basis of his expected harm and benefits under that principle" (Reibetanz 1998, 303–4).

It is not clear, however, why we must be driven to discount the complaint of anyone who is harmed by the improbability that he in particular would be harmed when we lack knowledge that anyone would be harmed. Suppose that there is a high chance—say a 95% chance—that one person would be killed if we act on a given principle, and a 5% chance that nobody would be killed, yet any given person would have only a 1 in 40 million chance of being killed. To illustrate this possibility, we can imagine a scenario that is identical to *Sacrifice Unknown Life (wheel)* except that there are now 38 million Californians rather than 40 million Californians underneath the roulette wheel. The wheel, however, still contains 40 million slots, a consequence of which is that two million of these slots do not lead to anyone's death. Rather, they lead to two million uninhabited patches of land in the Mojave Desert. Why should the fact that we do not know, since there is merely a 95% chance, that anyone at all would be killed prompt us to sharply discount the complaint of anyone who would die by the great improbability that he in particular would die, whereas when we are sure that somebody would die, we give that unknown person a non-discounted complaint that is just as large as the harm of premature death he would suffer? Reibetanz's proposal is unmotivated by the considerations she offers in its favor.

To be sure, we do not know that anyone would end up with a complaint of premature death in this scenario, but we are 95% certain that someone would end up with such a complaint. I propose that, rather than following Reibetanz's advice, we should instead posit a complaint of premature death in this scenario, where this complaint is discounted in a manner that tracks the probability that someone would suffer this fate. When applied to the scenario in question, there would be the following case against being exposed to risk. There is a 95% chance that someone would be killed as the result of such exposure, and a 5% chance that nobody would be killed. Since the risk of death falls short of certainty, we should not treat this scenario as identical to *Sacrifice Unknown Life (wheel)*, in which it is certain that someone would be killed. We should surely prefer the imposition of a 95% chance that one person would die over the imposition of a 100% chance that one person would die. Nevertheless, we should treat the former imposition as nearly as bad as the imposition of a certainty of death. We should register a strong complaint on behalf of that one victim, whoever in particular he may end up being, who is 95% certain to exist.[10] But we should discount this complaint by 5% to reflect the chance that nobody would suffer any harm.

---

[10] As before, this person need not be a determinate Californian.

There are circumstances in which my proposal that we discount a complaint against suffering harm by the chance that *someone* would actually suffer such harm converges on the more familiar proposal that we discount a person's complaint against suffering harm by the chance that *he* would suffer such harm. They converge when only one person, rather than a population of people, is subjected to an objective risk of harm. If, for example, there is only one gun, pointed at one Californian, then he alone suffers a 1 in 40 million risk of being killed, and the low risk that he would be killed is identical to the low risk that anyone would be killed. When, however, populations rather than just single individuals are subjected to risks of harm, and the risk that any particular individual would suffer harm therefore diverges from the risk that someone would suffer harm, my proposal is that harms should be more modestly discounted by the latter probability that someone would suffer harm rather than the former, lower probability, for any particular person, that he would suffer harm.

Even when we discount harms more modestly in this manner, perhaps it will still be possible to justify the flights over Andaman Islanders that I mentioned in section 1.[11] To test this hypothesis, let us not discount all the way down to the vanishingly small probability, for each islander, that he or she in particular will be the victim of a falling airplane. Rather, let us discount down to the probability that an Andaman Islander will be killed in this fashion. That latter probability will be higher than the former. But perhaps it is not so much higher as to render flights over the Andaman Islands impermissible. To be sure, the likelihood that someone in the world will be struck and killed by a falling plane within, say, the next 20 years approaches 100%. Nevertheless, the likelihood that at least one Andaman Islander will meet such a death is much lower. When we discount by this low likelihood, perhaps the discounted complaint is not so great as to stand in the way of flights over the Andaman Islands. The aggregate benefits of air travel to others might be morally relevant to, and sufficiently great to outweigh, a complaint, even of death, that has been discounted to that extent.

5.

In the previous section, I proposed that we should discount a complaint against suffering harm by the chance that someone would actually suffer such harm. I shall now apply my proposal to what has come to be known as the question of how the numbers should count. More precisely, I shall explore the moral significance of the fact that some number of individuals greater than one would

---

[11] See pp. 78–79, and recall the qualification in n. 3.

or might be killed as the result of risky activities. I shall begin by noting that the imposition on each of the risk of being killed in *Sacrifice Unknown Number of Lives (guns)* is, in the following important respect, harder to justify than the imposition on each of the risk of being killed in *Sacrifice Unknown Life (wheel)*: whereas it is certain that no more than one person would be killed in *Sacrifice Unknown Life (wheel)*, there is some chance that more than one person would be killed in *Sacrifice Unknown Number of Lives (guns)*. We must also bear in mind that there is the following respect in which *Sacrifice Unknown Number of Lives (guns)* is easier to justify than *Sacrifice Unknown Life (wheel)*: there is some chance—in fact, a 37% chance—that nobody would be killed in *Sacrifice Unknown Number of Lives (guns)*, whereas there is no chance that nobody would be killed in *Sacrifice Unknown Life (wheel)*. Moreover, the chances that more than one, and that fewer than one, would be killed in *Sacrifice Unknown Number of Lives (guns)* morally balance each other out in the following respect: if we were to expose a very large number of different populations containing 40 million individuals to the risks of *Sacrifice Unknown Number of Lives (guns)*, the average number of deaths per population of 40 million would converge on one death. It is, I think, reasonable to draw the conclusion that it is, all things considered, *just as hard* to justify the imposition of risk in *Sacrifice Unknown Life (wheel)* as it is to justify the imposition of risk in *Sacrifice Unknown Number of Lives (guns)*.[12]

More generally, it is reasonable to conclude that it is, other things equal, not any harder to justify a scenario in which some number of people would be subjected to a chance p of a given harm, where p is greater than zero and less than 100%, and someone would be certain to suffer this harm, than it is to justify a scenario in which the same number of people would be subjected to the same chance p of an equally great harm, yet there is some chance that nobody would be harmed.[13] It is no harder to justify, as that chance that nobody would

---

[12] Would I also say the same of a course of action that would kill A if a coin lands heads and kill B if the coin lands tails, when compared with an alternative course of action that would kill both A and B if a coin lands heads and kill neither if the coin lands tails? Namely, would I say that the former course of action is just as hard to justify as the latter? Yes, save for the badness of the inequality in the first scenario, which is absent in the second.

[13] This needs to be qualified to take account of the following: Since the former involves ex post inequality, and the latter does not, a two-person case with inversely correlated risks—heads A dies and B lives, tails B dies and A lives—is harder to justify than a two-person case with perfectly correlated risks—heads both A and B die, tails both A and B live (see Otsuka and Voorhoeve 2009, 196–98). Similarly, in *Sacrifice Unknown Life (wheel)*, we know that there would be the ex post inequality of one person dying, whereas everyone else lives, whereas in *Sacrifice Unknown Number of Lives (guns)*, we know that there is a 37% chance that there would be no ex post inequality, as that is the chance that nobody would die. That is counterbalanced by a chance that more than one would die, but the latter is not obviously worse, from the point of view of ex post inequality, than a scenario in which one would die for certain. This difference obtains so long as we consider the ex post inequalities in isolation from other inequalities. If, however, we do not, then this difference goes away. (See last paragraph of this section.)

be harmed will be morally balanced out by a chance that more than one person would be harmed in the manner described above. Such moral balancing will obtain so long as we are willing to embrace the following *constant marginal disvalue claim* that the moral significance of the difference between n versus $n + 1$ individuals suffering a given harm is the same, for any whole number n, including the number zero.

When, in accordance with this constant marginal disvalue claim, we allow for the augmenting of the combined force of any complaints against a risky course of action by the probability that more than one individual would suffer a given harm as well as the discounting of complaints by the probability that less than one individual would suffer this harm, such augmenting and discounting is nothing more than sensitivity to the probability that this or that number of individuals would end up suffering a given harm in those cases in which we do not know in advance how many this would be. What becomes relevant is simply the expected number who would suffer this harm under a given course of action. That is how the numbers count in the scenarios under discussion in this chapter.

Should we embrace this constant marginal disvalue claim? One might argue that we should not, on grounds that there is special significance to the fact that nobody as opposed to somebody would suffer a given harm as the result of a given risky course of action, where this significance exceeds the significance of the fact that some positive whole number versus that number plus one would suffer this harm. This might seem especially plausible in the case of very large numbers. Is the moral significance of the fact that 1,000,001 rather than 1,000,000 would die as the result of some risky course of action really just as great as the significance of the fact that one person would die rather than nobody as the result of another risky course of action? Some might deny this moral equivalence on the Stalinist grounds that "a single death is a tragedy; a million deaths is a statistic."[14] Presumably one who thinks this would also regard 1,000,001 deaths as a statistic. The problem with this line of thinking is that death number 1,000,001 is also a single death and tragedy for the person who suffers it. It is made no less tragic for him by the fact that one million others have also died. Why, in the light of this observation, is it of any special moral significance that a given risky course of action might turn out to impose no harms whatsoever on anybody? Note that this will be against a background of some number of harms that have already occurred due to risky activity more generally. So it will not, from a wider perspective, involve the possibility of no harm whatsoever. It will probably also be against the background of some number of harms that have already occurred due to risky activity in the past by the very same governmental agency that is now

---

[14] This assertion has been widely, though perhaps apocryphally, attributed to Joseph Stalin.

contemplating what to do. In the light of these facts, we should, I think, embrace the constant marginal disvalue claim.

6.

Drawing the above strands of argument together, it emerges from this discussion that there is little if any moral significance to the distinction between identified and nonidentified victims. The case for preventing the greater harm is not undermined when—as in the case of *Sacrifice Unknown Life (dust)*—the lack of knowledge of the identity of a victim is simply a matter of our ignorance of who this person would be, rather than of objective risks this person would share with others. Even when—as in the case of *Sacrifice Unknown Life (wheel)*—the lack of knowledge of the identity of a victim is explained by the fact that many would face the same objective and indeterministic risk of harm, that fact hardly undermines the case for preventing the greater harm. It hardly undermines this case even when the identity of the victim is, in principle, unknowable, because there is no fact of the matter who he would be, given the openness of counterfactuals. When, moreover, neither the number nor the identity (or identities) of would-be victim(s) is known—as in the case of *Sacrifice Unknown Number of Lives (guns)*—that fact does not undermine the case for preventing the greatest expected harm rather than exhibiting a preference for identified victims.

Acknowledgments

I have presented versions of this chapter at the Australian National University, Harvard, the London School of Economics, Macquarie University, Queen's University Belfast, Queen's University at Kingston, Trinity College Dublin, University College London, University of California, Riverside, and the Universities of Copenhagen, Gothenburg, Hull, Manchester, Missouri, Oxford, Pavia, Sheffield, Toronto, and Vermont. I thank the members of the audiences for their comments. I would also like to thank Paul Weirich, Matthew Adler, Geoffrey Brennan, Thomas Dougherty, Nir Eyal, Cécile Fabre, Johann Frick, Barbara Fried, Caspar Hare, Elizabeth Harman, Ian Phillips, Kenneth Simons, Thomas Porter Sinclair, Peter Vallentyne, Alex Voorhoeve, and the late G. A. Cohen for their comments.

References

Adler, Matthew. 2003. "Risk, Death and Harm: The Normative Foundations of Risk Regulation." *Minnesota Law Review* 87: 1293–445.

Hare, Caspar. 2012. "Obligations to Merely Statistical People." *Journal of Philosophy* 109: 378–90.
Kamm, F. M. 1993. *Morality, Mortality*. Vol. 1. Oxford: Oxford University Press.
Otsuka, M., and A. Voorhoeve. 2009. "Why It Matters That Some Are Worse Off Than Others: An Argument against the Priority View." *Philosophy and Public Affairs* 37: 171–99.
Reibetanz, Sophia. 1998. "Contractualism and Aggregation." *Ethics* 108: 296–311.
Scanlon, T. M. 1998. *What We Owe to Each Other*. Cambridge, MA: Harvard University Press.

6 }

Concentrated Risk, the Coventry Blitz, Chamberlain's Cancer

Nir Eyal

1. Background

The Coventry Blitz attack of November 14, 1940, sowed urban destruction on a scale previously unimaginable in Britain. Bomb shock and fire damaged two out of every three buildings in the city, leveling more than 4,000. Overnight, hundreds of Coventry inhabitants were killed and hundreds were injured (Foot 2002; Dear and Foot 2002; Gilbert 1992, 684; BBC 2013).

A 1974 book claimed that Winston Churchill knew in advance about the looming aerial attack on Coventry. Intercepted German radio messages, encrypted with the German Enigma cipher machine, were decrypted by British intelligence and revealed the Coventry Blitz plan. But Churchill allegedly decided to do nothing. Any defensive measure would have alerted the Germans that their cipher had been broken, with greater impact on the British war effort and a higher overall British death toll (Winterbotham 1975).

The claim that Coventry was sacrificed for the code has been repeated many times, typically with a critical valence. For example, five years ago, a play performed in Coventry suggested that "Churchill, forewarned of the German attack, deliberately sacrificed the citizens of Coventry"; that suggestion was immediately understood as an "accusation" of some "gravity"— an "incendiary" suggestion (Billington 2008; Gardner 2008).

The oft-repeated claim turns out to be a myth, historians now agree. For example, the decoding of the Enigma cipher did not name only Coventry as a potential target for a Blitz attack, so Churchill did not know in advance which city would be attacked, only that one would be attacked. If anything, his overall intelligence indicated, and he believed, that that city would be London.[1]

---

[1] Additionally, Churchill's sole specific evidence about Coventry came from an investigation of a seized German pilot and not from the decoding of the Enigma cipher, so acting to defend Coventry

But my interest in this event is not historical. What intrigues me is our moral intuition about this case—real or, as it turns out, mythical. It is interesting that most people feel that if the claim were correct, then Churchill or his apologists would have to defend him from a potentially grave "accusation." At least, many feel, his decision would not have been a morally trivial one, a matter of accurate calculation of net expected deaths (perhaps after discounting future deaths somewhat, simply because they would occur later). Initially there seems to be more to the ethics of this than whether or not such a decision would in fact promote utility and save lives on balance. A small gain in the prospect of properly weighted life-saving, we initially want to say, would not be enough to justify sacrificing Coventrians.

This intuition is not about doing versus allowing—it was the Germans, and not Churchill, who actively bombed Coventry. Nor is it about intending versus merely foreseeing—the myth has Churchill sacrifice Coventry as a mere foreseen side effect of hiding intelligence from the Germans and thereby winning the war.[2] Nor is the intuition about special fiduciary obligations toward the inhabitants of Coventry—any special fiduciary obligations that Churchill might have had toward Coventrians he also had toward other British inhabitants. Nor is the intuition one about outcome inequality. Coventrian casualties would have introduced inequality between the sorry fates of some who would die prematurely and the happier lots of the living, but so would any war casualty. What exactly would be wrong, then, about a decision to sacrifice Coventrians—passively—for the sake of minimizing the number of overall deaths?

When a named person or a group, such as the inhabitants of Coventry, is identified as being at elevated risk, we often feel that this is unfair and that other things being equal, they command priority for protective measures. Abandoning them to elevated risk for the sake of collective utility or its more equal distribution is problematic, we are inclined to say. Other things being equal, their abandonment would remain a wrong-making feature of our policy. Fairness demands "risk pooling"—redistributing risk more equally. Or so common-sense morality assumes.

Recently, Norman Daniels, Michael Otsuka, and Johann Frick have used this way of thinking in an attempt to explain why people identified as

---

could not have possibly threatened the decoding coup. Some special defenses for Coventry, which Churchill may have considered adequate, had been put in place earlier that month. Finally, when at three o'clock in the afternoon, a few hours before the attack, the Royal Air Force realized that the attack would take place that night in Coventry, measures to defend the city were taken immediately—and largely foundered (Hinsley 1979, 316–18 and appendix 9; Calvocoressi 1980, 76; Gilbert 1992, 683–84; Kimball 1998, 351 n. 2; Edgerton 2011, 68–69; Manchester and Reid 2012, 215–17). While these individually sufficient refutations might not all be mutually compatible, some clearly stand.

[2] Compare another myth, according to which Churchill sacrificed Coventry intentionally, and not merely as a side effect—so that photos of the destruction on front pages of American newspapers would hasten American entry in the war (Gardner 2008).

high-risk—in our example, the population of Coventry—command some moral priority (Daniels 2012; Daniels, in this volume; Otsuka 2011; Frick 2010). While curbing the overall death toll matters, curbing elevated risks to some—risks that, as Daniels puts it, are "concentrated" in some people and populations more than in others—also matters (and see a similar position in Sher 1980, 203; Broome 1990).

An elegant illustration of this philosophical position on the concentration of risk is found in Daniels's contribution to this volume:

> Suppose we have only five tablets of a medicine that can be used either as an effective treatment for a disease (Treatment), provided that all five tablets are given, or that can be given in one-tablet doses to people exposed to the disease, where it acts as an effective vaccination (Vaccination). Without vaccination, one of the five exposed people will contract the disease and then die. That is, each has a 20% chance of contracting the disease and dying once exposed.
>
> *Treatment*: Alice has the disease. We can give her the whole dose.
>
> *Vaccination*: Betty, Cathy, Dolly, Ellie, and Fannie have been exposed to Alice. We can vaccinate all of them with one-fifth of the dose we can give Alice.
>
> ... Does the concentration of risk in the Treatment Case matter morally? Do we have a greater obligation to treat or vaccinate?
>
> I believe we have a stronger obligation to treat Alice than to vaccinate the five others. (Daniels, in this volume).

Although later in his chapter Daniels clarifies that his ultimate position is relatively weak—applied to this case, perhaps it is only that there is reasonable disagreement on whether the obligation to treat Alice is stronger—his position in the quoted passage is strong and, I find, especially interesting: we "have a stronger obligation to treat Alice than to vaccinate the five others." Daniels also explains that this obligation is a matter of fairness toward the worse off:

> To see the issue of distributive fairness that is at work here, consider why Alice arguably has the stronger claim on assistance: she is worse off than the other five at the point of deliberation about how to use the medicine. She faces certain death if nothing is done or if others get the vaccination, whereas they face "only" a 20% chance of death if nothing is done or if Alice is rescued. Since her claim on assistance is stronger, it would be unfair to her to favor the others, who have weaker claims. (Daniels, in this volume)

The present chapter focuses on the strong position that I identify in these passages. Do we "have a stronger obligation to treat Alice than to vaccinate the five others"? And do we have that obligation because risk concentration lends claims of "distributive" fairness to those at concentrated risk—say, because they count as worse off? Does the distribution of risk and chance count intrinsically as a matter of fairness—as Broome, Daniels, Frick, Otsuka, and Sher seem to hold?

I shall argue that we lack inherent duties to prioritize those at concentrated risk as a matter of distributive fairness. Alice, for example, does not count as worse off. That said, we may have instrumental or other indirect reasons to prioritize. Churchill, for example, might have had instrumental or indirect reasons against sacrificing Coventrians even if sacrificing them would save more lives by maintaining the Enigma deciphering achievement. Perhaps sacrificing Coventrians would have looked so cruel if discovered that doing so gambled too much on Britons' reputation for solidarity and compassion and perhaps on their willingness to act compassionately in the long run. Perhaps if Churchill were concerned enough about the latter danger, he would have schooled himself to refuse to sacrifice anyone in the first place. But that would still not mean that in November 1940, Churchill had noninstrumental, nonderivative reasons to prioritize Coventrians—that other things being equal, they had stronger claims on him for assistance than Britons who were not individually at high risk. I shall argue that in terms of its inherent worth and nonderivative rightness, letting some people or populations stay at concentrated risk, greater risk than others face, remains fair. Equality is fairer than inequality, but that ought to mean equality of bad and good outcomes, not equality of risks and good prospects.

I shall distinguish between two different things that risk, and hence risk concentration, can mean in this setting (in the next section). This will put us in a better position to see that risk concentration does not matter intrinsically on either interpretation. Risk concentration can remain fair when risk is understood in epistemic terms (the following three sections). And it can remain fair when risk is understood in nonepistemic terms (final section). The conclusion is that there is nothing inherently unfair about risk concentration.

2. What Does Risk Concentration Mean?

It so happens that hours before the Coventry Blitz, Churchill was among the pallbearers at Neville Chamberlain's funeral. Chamberlain had long enjoyed good health, but on July 29 that year he entered hospital for surgery. The surgeons discovered that he was suffering from terminal bowel cancer, but they concealed it from him, telling him that he would not require further surgery. Chamberlain left hospital thinking that he was all right. A little over three months later, he died of bowel cancer, in excruciating pain (Gilbert 1992, 683; Self 2006, 442–43).

On the morning after the operation, I imagine an optimistic Chamberlain. He must have continued to feel pain, but may have considered it to be a passing postoperative unpleasantness. A fortnight past the operation he wrote a friend that he expected to "go forward like a two year old now" (Self 2006, 443). Let us ask: The morning after the operation, was Chamberlain at concentrated risk of death in the succeeding months?

The answer depends on what we mean by "risk." If we asked Chamberlain or investigated the best evidence he possessed, the answer would be that, thanks to a successful surgery, he now faced a low risk of imminent death (let us assume he had strong reason to suspect that the surgeons would not lie about certain death to him, a senior cabinet minister in the midst of war). On that interpretation of risk, Chamberlain was probably free from cancer, not at all facing a concentrated risk of death within months. Objectively, however, the advanced tumor continued to be there. In a nonepistemic sense, notwithstanding Chamberlain's optimism and the evidence available to him, he continued to be at high risk of impending death from cancer.

Both epistemic (or subjective) and nonepistemic (or objective) interpretations of risk come in different stripes. Epistemic interpretations vary according to whether what fixes them is the evidence available to the agent, her actual belief, or still other epistemic variables; and for different agents.

Nonepistemic interpretations, namely ones that do not fix risk by any doxastic state, also have subspecies. We will focus on the simplest one—the nonepistemic interpretation in which Chamberlain's advanced cancer stage that morning put him at very high risk. Objectively—regardless of what he believed or had evidence for, Chamberlain was that morning very likely to die within a year. One way to cash out that objective interpretation of Chamberlain's "risk" of cancer death surrounds frequency: roughly that among the finite set of people who had earlier had the same type of cancer, a high frequency had died soon thereafter. Another way to cash out that objective interpretation focuses on the slightly different notion of propensity: roughly, that people at a similar physical state due to cancer had a strong propensity or disposition to die within a year. This variance of nonepistemic senses of risk is immaterial to our purposes.[3]

This categorization dovetails with the bulk of literature on interpretations of probability and risk in general (Hájek 2012; Hansson 2012; Hacking 2006, 11–18; Oberdiek 2009, 369–70; Schaffer 2007, 136–39) and on interpretations of risk concentration in particular (Sher 1980; Adler 2003, 1297; Otsuka, in this

---

[3] There is also a third, "philosophers'," nonepistemic sense or account of risk, according to which, simply because a little over three months later Chamberlain was dead, and because in a deterministic world, all the elementary particles that would make this the case were in place that morning and already determined all future events, then (assuming ours is a deterministic world and setting aside some philosophical complications), on the morning after the operation, Chamberlain was already at maximal risk of dying within a year. His probability of impending death was not just close to 1, it was 1. What I say below about nonepistemic risk applies to this "philosophers'" nonepistemic interpretation as well.

volume, n. 6). Whether risk is concentrated in you depends on what notion of risk is being used.

The rest of this chapter uses this categorization to bolster the point that risk concentration does not inherently give rise to fair claims to protective resources, not even when other things are equal. Sometimes risk concentration is high but intuitively there is no unfairness to speak of and no urgency to pool that risk. This becomes apparent once we unbundle the notion of risk, looking separately at epistemic and nonepistemic risks.

3. Epistemic Risk Concentration

Let us begin by plugging epistemic notions of risk into the claim that Churchill's (mythical) decision to sacrifice Coventrians and cut overall deaths by a small number was unfair and inherently wrong. Epistemic risk focuses on beliefs or evidence. We shall focus on Churchill's beliefs and evidence. Another subspecies of epistemic risk would focus on the risks as assessed by others, such as Coventrians and the evidence available to them. But according to Coventrians' beliefs and evidence on the eve of the attack, the risk they faced was commensurate with that of other Britons. That interpretation of risk is a nonstarter for defending the position that Coventrians were at unfairly high risk. So it is more promising to focus on Churchill's doxastic states. Had Churchill decided to sacrifice Coventrians for the war effort, would that treat them unfairly by failing to protect them from what his beliefs and best evidence suggested is concentrated risk? Would he be acting unfairly even if objectively, Coventrians were not at elevated risk, for example, if the attack was set to launch on another British city?

Anyone making this claim would immediately face the following challenge. Why focus on what is merely epistemic—in Churchill's mind or in his initial evidence only and not in the world "itself"? Why would Churchill's potentially false beliefs and misleading evidence on whether the Germans would descend on Coventry matter more to fairness than Chamberlain's false beliefs and misleading evidence on the advance of disease mattered to his survival?

4. Against an "Equal Concern" Answer to the Challenge

Several philosophers who take epistemic risk seriously answer that challenge by citing the value of equal concern, the foremost "sovereign virtue" according to Dworkinians and proponents of social equality. As they explain, abandoning someone to more risk than you would abandon others to usually shows unequal or inadequate concern. When racist or favoritist allocators who lack equal concern allocate what they take to be the risks and the prospects unequally, that is already unfair, even when their attempts to allocate risks in objectively unequal portions founder (Wasserman 1996, 39). In fact, this is why "a payoff condition that [secured] epistemic equiprobability might well express an equal commitment to each claimant [especially] emphatically" (39). In Daniels's words, "If an identified victim faces a high risk of death, *concern* to avoid her loss will lead to willingness to pay an amount that is much greater than what people are willing to pay to save an equivalent number of statistical lives spread over a broader population" (Daniels, in this volume, emphasis added).

Equal epistemic chance can also be associated with impartiality and equal concern on the negative ground of what epistemic equiprobability protects against: "The fact that the allocator has no idea whether the coin will land Heads or Tails ensures that she cannot act partially and show favour for one party over another" (Otsuka 2011; see also Wasserman 1996, 31; compare Kaplow and Shavell 2001, 285).[4] Wasserman sometimes writes that coin flipping and epistemic equiprobability are a helpful "prophylaxis" against unequal concern.

But consider how an equal-concern-based answer to the challenge would work in Churchill's case. As it turns out, some people who believe that Churchill sacrificed Coventry also cast doubt on his equal concern for Coventrians. They wonder whether Churchill, a conservative aristocrat, might have been a little too ready to sacrifice an industrial Midlands town with many Communists who resisted his war efforts. The writer whose play had Churchill knowingly sacrifice Coventry told an interviewer, "I can't help thinking that, if the intelligence had said that Oxford or Cambridge or the W1 postal districts of London were the target, then the decision would have been different" (Gardner 2008). Undoubtedly, abandoning an identified person or group to concentrated risk can leave us wondering about the adequacy or equality of the allocator's concern for them. But clearly this cannot make every instance of concentrated risk unfair. Not every allocator who knowingly leaves someone at concentrated risk for whatever purpose does so out of low or lesser concern for that person. The allocator may have other motives such as saving more lives, increasing outcome equality, or military fanaticism. What psychologically drives or enables his or her decision need not include racism, favoritism, or anything of the sort. Whether or not the playwright's suspicion of Churchill is true, there is no case for tarnishing all allocators past, present, and future, who decide to abandon relatively identified victims to concentrated risk, as allegedly having done so

---

[4] Alex Voorhoeve made an interesting suggestion on this: "This is a bad argument, since it doesn't help in the following scenario:*Option 1*—Ann lives and Bob dies (both for sure); *Option 2*—Heads: Ann dies, Bob lives; Tails: Ann lives, Bob dies. Here, someone partial to Bob will favour Option 2 (equal chances), because it is the best he can do for Bob. So equal chances doesn't always express impartial concern."

out of lesser concern for them. Many will have done so out of other good or bad motives. A computer programmed to be equally mindful of interests and decide purely in the light of cost-effectiveness standards might give different people unequal chances. Even if something is necessarily wrong in such decisions, that something cannot be the alleged wrongfulness of acting out of unequal concern (unless "equal concern" means something different than what Sher, Wasserman, Daniels, Otsuka, and others have discussed—we could assess it once the alternate notion is laid out fully).

Take what actually happened before the Coventry Blitz. Several hours earlier, Churchill did decide to place one city at concentrated epistemic risk, but that city was one whose inhabitants he clearly valued. That city was London, and one inhabitant whom he believed would encounter elevated mortal risk was himself:

> On November 14 Churchill . . . read the most recent Air Intelligence estimate of forthcoming German bomber targets. It seemed almost certain that a heavy raid was in prospect that very night. Its target was not yet known; but several earlier reports had suggested that the next big raid would be on London. Churchill at once told his driver to turn round and take him back to Downing Street. He was not going to spend the night "peacefully in the country," he told the Private Secretary [who later recounted this], "while the metropolis was under heavy attack." On returning to Downing Street to await the raid on London, Churchill gave instructions for the women members of his staff to be sent home. Later he sent two of his Private Secretaries to a deep air-raid shelter in Piccadilly with the words "You are too young to die." He then waited impatiently for the raid to begin . . . on the Air Ministry roof. (Gilbert 1992, 863–64).

Imagine that Churchill could have done more to defend London but instead abandoned it in order to cut war deaths by a small number.[5] Then Churchill put Londoners at concentrated epistemic risk from his viewpoint. But surely it does not follow that he had sweeping low concern for all those he was placing at risk. Any account of his motives must be more subtle, because Churchill knew that he was placing himself and some who were near and dear to him at risk.

What is true is only that sometimes, exposing identified people to concentrated risk, even for an otherwise good reason, initially appears as though it must stem from lower concern for them, especially when these people had been persistent

---

[5] Here is how that might play out. Another mythical conspiracy depicts Churchill's goal in sacrificing Coventry as hastening America's entry in the war. Photos of the burned-out ruins of Coventry's medieval cathedral on American newspaper front pages may have accomplished that (Gardner 2008). Likewise, we may imagine Churchill hoping for photos of Westminster Abbey lying in ruins, or his own burned corpse on the Air Ministry roof, to sway America to enter the war.

victims of low concern before the decision took place or before it becomes publicly known. The 1974 allegations about the sacrifice of Coventry may have been a case in point, for reasons that had nothing to do with Churchill's motives. As the playwright admits, "The rumours came at a time when the city was no longer feeling confident about itself. Factories were closing down. It made us wonder whether the city had been considered expendable" (Gardner 2008).

My aim is not to get Churchill completely off the moral hook. There can be instrumental reasons to avoid even the appearance of partiality—by equalizing risk exposure. My own, philosophical point is that these reasons are merely contingent, not reasons of fairness to the worse off in terms of risk exposure—which would have been inherent to the situation. Had the attack been planned for the W1 district of London and the risk allocator, Churchill, were widely known to have the highest concern for those at risk, these instrumental reasons would not be there. It is true that perspicuously equalizing epistemic risk, say, by making risk-distribution decisions only by flipping an even coin between equal prospects, can help stem any potential for (the appearance of) partiality. But it is philosophically crude to confuse this typical usefulness of a coin toss with intrinsically and invariably worthy equal concern. For one thing, when it is plain that the allocator cares a lot for identified victims and would never discriminate against them, further prophylaxis against (suspicion of) partiality serves no purpose.

5. Against Other Answers to the Challenge

Some friends of epistemic risk pooling may now attempt to lend it other justificatory foundations, instead of the value of equal concern. But postulating a duty to pool epistemic risk generates absurdities no matter what concrete foundation is ascribed to that duty.

For instance, imagine that the Battle of Britain is on, and that you are staffing a tall power station in the center of a densely populated British city. A Blitz raid begins. As Luftwaffe planes start dropping shells and buildings catch fire, you look out of your window and notice a streetlamp that was erroneously left undimmed. A nearby house and its residents are therefore at concentrated risk for mortal attacks, because German pilots used lights as convenient targets. You control the power system and could turn off the streetlight. There would be considerable financial cost, but the house residents' lives might be saved, and you judge the cost to be well worth the high chance of saving lives. Then, however, you have a second thought: What would turning the light off accomplish? German bombs are already pounding your densely populated city (which has no empty lots). If this house is spared, another house will not be. Flicking the lights off for the sake of that house's residents will only reallocate objective danger. It will not reduce it. Is it really something that you have strong moral reason to do, reason enough to justify considerable financial cost?

Had you had strong reason to redistribute all concentrated epistemic risk from your current viewpoint—to "pool" that epistemic risk—it would have been morally urgent to turn the streetlight off, even at some financial cost. After all, to do so would ward off concentrated epistemic risk. Admittedly it would jeopardize an unknown other house's residents but, because it would remain unknown to you who your victims would be, equality of epistemic risk would increase and the worse off in terms of epistemic risk would be prioritized in its distribution. As far as epistemic risk goes, turning the light off would be like substituting a very uneven coin by an even one. While objectively, risks would be shifted around with no equalization or priority to the worse off, epistemically, risk distribution would become more equal.[6]

But that is ridiculous. Quite clearly, switching the light off is pointless; the diffusion of sheer epistemic risk does not improve fairness (or make you a better person). In fact, the equality (or priority) of epistemic risk from your current viewpoint would likewise increase if turning this streetlight off turned on another one in front of another house in town, currently unknown to you, a moment later; and if turning that light off would a moment later turn on another, and so forth. As in musical chairs, this process could continue until it was time to stop. At that point, the same number of people would die as originally predicted, with some financial waste.

I guess some die-hard epistemic-risk redistributors might insist, despite this waste, that our deontic duty remains that of reallocating epistemic risk more equitably. After all, who ever said that acting right repeatedly would necessarily lead to the best outcomes? But if every switching off of a light trained you to switch off the next light faster, as well as training the system to switch on the next light faster, eventually reaching superhuman speeds, then this process of reallocating risk would never end (imagine that after a certain number of transactions the marginal financial cost of new ones would be nil). Would it even be logically consistent, then, to insist on our duty to keep redirecting risks? The following genuine Blitz era anecdote illustrates a similarly ridiculous process, with God as allocator:

> A London vicar asked a fellow occupant of his basement shelter whether she prayed when she heard a bomb falling. "Yes," she answered, "I pray, Oh God! Don't let it fall here." The vicar said, "But it's a bit rough on other people, if your prayer is granted and the thing drops, not on you, but on them." The woman replied, "I can't help that. They must say their prayers and push it further." (Hastings 2012, 93).

---

[6] This action to defend the identified house residents while putting others at risk might be seen as problematic only because it involves putting some at risk actively. However, dimming the light to prevent the bombers from taking aim at a house is best seen as defensive action. The destructive agency is still the responsibility of the bombers, not the defender.

To summarize, if persons epistemically known to be at elevated risk commanded even moderate priority over others, then it would have been important to turn off any streetlight currently on, and thereby save the inhabitants of the adjacent house, even at the expense of another house's inhabitants. But once the implications are fully laid out, the absurdity of assigning us such a duty becomes apparent. The lesson I draw from this, and from the failure to ground duties to redistribute epistemic risk in the value of equal concern, is that the concentration of epistemic risk in someone does not create duties of fairness to prioritize that person.

6. Nonepistemic Risk Concentration

It is tempting to conclude at this point that what fairness demands is the equalizing of nonepistemic risk. But the nonepistemic risk interpretation remains unsuccessful at clarifying why Churchill's decision to sacrifice Coventry (had he made one) would be wrong. Those historians according to whom Churchill knew enough about the German plans to tell that one British city was at high risk, but was unaware which,[7] assume that they thereby sufficiently exonerate Churchill from any accusation of unfair treatment of Coventrians. Precisely because historians are not moral philosophers, this tacit moral assumption is likelier to capture raw intuition than our own proclaimed assumptions are. We should let historians be our native speakers.

A colleague who preferred to remain unnamed initially objected to this, writing:

> I disagree. If Churchill knew that some British city would be attacked by the Luftwaffe that evening and had enough planes to defend all British cities ... then choosing not to stop the attack in order not to compromise the British deciphering operation at Bletchley Park would be morally problematic, even if this would lead to fewer deaths in the long run. One way of putting this is that Churchill would have sacrificed the inhabitants of one city (by failing to aid them) as the means to achieving a good, i.e. saving more lives in the future by not revealing the existence of the deciphering program. In this case, a harm is "causally upstream" from a good in a way that many non-consequentialists ... find problematic. The fact that Churchill did not know which city he was sacrificing seems

---

[7] For example, Churchill's biographer writes that although it had been clear that a big raid was looming, "for some days there had been conflicting indications about the target of the next big raid. Not only London, but also the Thames Valley, the Kent or Essex coasts, Coventry, and Birmingham, had each been mentioned as the possible target" (Gilbert 1992, 863). Johann Frick suggested to me that the many historians who press this point in defense of Churchill may mean simply that defending all these areas simultaneously would have been impossible. But Churchill could have helped all these areas to some degree, for instance by alerting the fire and ambulance services on the radio (Gardner 2008).

irrelevant to this assessment, as long as we assume that Churchill did have the option of protecting all British cities that night. (e-mail correspondence, September 26, 2011).

This colleague's position is eloquently phrased, but in a later conversation he changed his mind, and for good reason. Almost every major action of a leader in a just war has some causal impact on, among other things, which persons on his or her side are nonepistemically at risk. When the leader remains oblivious as to who these persons are, surely he cannot be expected to avoid acting. As an illustration, in 1940 Britain, many defensive or offensive measures, or even non-war-related policies, were likely to affect details of German decisions in the succeeding period, including decisions on which British towns to bomb next. There is a simple reason why British measures often had impact on German decisions and thus, objectively, on which Britons would come under concentrated nonepistemic risk. In order not to be too predictable to the enemy's military intelligence, German decision-makers allowed their own last-minute whims to determine details, such as which of several British cities to bomb next. Often in wartime, decision-makers defer actual detailed decisions till last minute and let arbitrary facts inform those details, for precisely that reason. Thus, anything affecting German decision-makers' thinking or mood at the relevant moment could have affected which Britons would die. Of course, Churchill and other British leaders had no way of telling how their actions would affect German decisions and hence, how objective risk would be distributed among Britons. But surely no otherwise-legitimate British measures were made wrong just because it was clear that objectively they had significant likelihood of affecting which Britons would die. The distribution of nonepistemic risk cannot affect what is unfair.[8]

We end by addressing a potential response to this conclusion. In one variant on the following classical case from Jonathan Glover, intuition initially seems to support focus on nonepistemic risk distribution:

> Anatol Rapoport recounts a case of air crews on high-risk missions in the Second World War. At a certain place, a pilot's chances of surviving his thirty bombing missions were only one in four. It was calculated that one-way missions, by reducing the fuel load, could increase the load of bombs, so that only half the pilots need fly. Selection would be by a lot, with half of the pilots escaping altogether and half going to certain death. On this system, fatalities would be halved, but it was not adopted.

---

[8] The colleague's point, "Churchill would have sacrificed the inhabitants of one city (by failing to aid them) as the means to achieving a good," may create the misleading impression that (according to the myth) the harm to Coventrians was Churchill's means to winning the war, and perhaps one he let happen intentionally. But as mentioned above, that harm was a mere side effect, not letting die as a means (for a case of the latter, see the Guinea Pig Case: Quinn 1989, 336; I thank Alex Voorhoeve for this reference).

Obviously there could be various reasons for not adopting the system, including the possibility that those who drew lots for certain death would not carry out the order. But there is also an extreme horror which most of us have at the thought of being in a position where we can see certain death ahead. The condemned cell is a lot of the awfulness of capital punishment. (Glover 1990, 212–13).

Consider a variant on this case. In the variant, both the pilots and everyone else would remain entirely oblivious as to who would go on a death mission and who would not. That is because, as all would know, a few of the pilots would be given enough fuel to return (a few more than half the planes would need to be sent). A secret lottery would then determine which planes would carry a full tank and which, extra bombs; another secret lottery would determine which pilot would fly which plane; and a firewall between the two secret lottery outcomes would ensure that, at takeoff, no one, neither pilot nor support staff, would know which pilots lacked the fuel to return. Pilots would discover that only in enemy airspace, when they would notice that they could release many bombs.

In this variant on Glover's case, all pilots would know in advance only that a few would return and most would not. That is what the staff would know too. All pilots would therefore face high epistemic risk from everyone's viewpoints, but none would be epistemically "condemned." That should take care of any special psychological horror from knowing that one will definitely die. And because this arrangement would decrease pilot casualties, epistemic risk from going through one's entire course of bombing missions would be smaller than under the conventional bombing method.

I suspect that most readers would remain very uneasy about this arrangement—possibly not much less than intuitively we are about the arrangement that Glover describes. Why? One account of our unease about both Glover's case and this variant is in terms of nonepistemic risk. Although everyone might be ignorant as to who exactly is being sent to his death, such arrangements might be thought to remain unfair toward those who, objectively, are being sent to their deaths. Even under the variant arrangement, as pilots took off, objectively it would already be determined that some stood no chance of returning. They would not know that they were condemned, any more than Chamberlain knew on the morning after his operation that he was bound to die soon. But their fates would be sealed. This might initially suggest that despite my claim above, concentrated nonepistemic risk is unfair.

But the reason why nonepistemic risk intuitively matters, either in Glover's case or in this variant, is not distributive fairness. Under either arrangement, the sufficient cause of death for any pilot who would board a plane without the fuel to return would be having abided by his own commanders' orders to set off on the mission. This might mean that, objectively, unless enemy fire caught them first, their killers would be their own commanders. The air force would actively kill its own pilots. Whether or not this holds real moral force, or just provides an adequate error theory, it easily accounts for our moral unease about either arrangement. There is no need to drag in distributive considerations.

Indeed, suppose that instead of a regular mechanized lottery, which some philosophers might consider nonchancy (see note 3 above), the air force used a (sci-fi) quantum lottery machine. That machine's genuinely indeterministic results would make it nonepistemically chancy who would take off without the fuel to return. Very clearly, no one would be "condemned" to death in advance. I believe that our judgments would remain pretty much the same. Sending pilots on certain-death missions would continue to feel highly objectionable. Our unease arises, then, whether or not it is clear that anyone is objectively "condemned." What generates that unease cannot be the alleged unfairness of a lopsided risk distribution (one in which some are "condemned" to death). It is something else, perhaps the likelihood that objectively, the pilot's killers could be his or her own commanders. In short, despite what this variation on Glover's case initially suggests, nonepistemic risk concentration does not undermine distributive fairness.

7. Conclusion

Epistemic or nonepistemic, high risk does not always strengthen our duty to assist a person or a group. Alice lacks a stronger claim to assistance than Betty, Cathy, and the others. There may remain any of a number of contingent, instrumental, and derivative reasons to prioritize those at concentrated risk. For example, many people may falsely perceive nonintervention as unfair and as expressive of disrespect toward Alice, and such perceptions may undermine political stability, Alice's sense of self-respect, or what have you. But philosophically, these matters remain contingent. What are not among the reasons to prioritize Alice—or, in Churchill's case, the residents of Coventry—are inherent claims to protection as a matter of fairness toward those at elevated risk.

Acknowledgments

The author is grateful to Johann Frick, Maya Jasanoff, Leah Price, Torbjörn Tännsjö, Alex Voorhoeve, Gerard Vong, audiences at the Frontiers of Political Philosophy 2010 workshop, the Swedish Congress of Philosophy 2013, the American Society for Bioethics and the Humanities 2013 conference, the University of Roskilde, and the Ethics Reading Group of the MIT Department of Philosophy for helpful comments.

References

Adler, Matthew D. 2003. "Risk, Death and Harm: The Normative Foundations of Risk Regulation." *Minnesota Law Review* 87: 1293–445.
BBC. 2013. "On This Day: 15 November, 1940: Germans Bomb Coventry to Destruction." Available from http://news.bbc.co.uk/onthisday/hi/dates/stories/november/15/newsid_3522000/3522785.stm.
Billington, Michael. 2008. "One Night in November." *The Guardian*, March 12.
Broome, John. 1990. "Fairness." *Proceedings of the Aristotelian Society* 91: 87–101.
Calvocoressi, Peter. 1980. *Top Secret Ultra*. New York: Pantheon Books.
Daniels, Norman. 2012. "Reasonable Disagreement about Identified vs. Statistical Victims." *Hastings Center Report* 42 (1): 35–45.
Dear, I. C. B., and M. R. D. Foot. 2002. "Coventry." In *The Oxford Companion to World War II*, edited by I. C. B. Dear and M. R. D. Foot, 213. New York: Oxford University Press.
Edgerton, David. 2011. *Britain's War Machine: Weapons, Resources, and Experts in the Second World War*. New York: Oxford University Press.
Foot, M. R. D. 2002. "Atrocities." In *The Oxford Companion to World War II*, edited by I. C. B. Dear and M. R. D. Foot, 59–60. New York: Oxford University Press.
Frick, Johann. 2010. "Health Resource Allocation behind a Natural Veil of Ignorance." Draft.
Gardner, Lyn. 2008. "The Ultimate Sacrifice." *The Guardian*, March 3.
Gilbert, Martin. 1992. *Churchill: A Life*. New York: Holt Paperbacks.
Glover, Jonathan. 1990. *Causing Death and Saving Lives*. London: Penguin.
Hacking, Ian. 2006. *The Emergence of Probability: A Philosophical Study of Early Ideas about Probability, Induction, and Statistical Inference*. 2d ed. New York: Cambridge University Press.
Hájek, Alan. 2012. "Interpretations of Probability." In *Stanford Encyclopedia of Philosophy* (Winter 2012 ed.), edited by Edward N. Zalta.
Hansson, Sven Ove. 2012. "Risk." In *Stanford Encyclopedia of Philosophy* (Winter 2012 ed.), edited by Edward N. Zalta.
Hastings, Max. 2012. *Inferno: The World at War, 1939–1945*. Reprint ed. New York: Vintage.
Hinsley, F. H. 1979. *British Intelligence in the Second World War: Its Influence on Strategy and Operations*. Vol. 1. Cambridge: Cambridge University Press.
Kaplow, Louis, and Steven Shavell. 2001. "Any Non-welfarist Method of Policy Assessment Violates the Pareto Principle." *Journal of Political Economy* 109 (2): 281–86.
Kimball, Warren F. 1998. *Forged in War: Roosevelt, Churchill, and the Second World War*. New York: Harper Perennial.
Manchester, William, and Paul Reid. 2012. *The Last Lion: Winston Spencer Churchill. Defender of the Realm, 1940–1965*. New York: Little, Brown.
Oberdiek, John. 2009. "Towards a Right against Risking." *Law and Philosophy* 28 (4): 367–92. doi:10.1007/s10982-008-9039-5.
Otsuka, Michael. 2011. ""The Fairness of Equal Chances." Draft.
Quinn, Warren S. 1989. "Actions, Intentions and Consequences: The Doctrine of Double Effect." *Philosophy and Public Affairs* 18 (4): 334–51.
Schaffer, Jonathan. 2007. "Deterministic Chance?" *British Journal for the Philosophy of Science* 58: 113–40.

Self, Robert. 2006. *Neville Chamberlain: A Biography*. Aldershot: Ashgate.
Sher, George. 1980. "What Makes a Lottery Fair?" *Nous* 14 (2): 203–16.
Wasserman, David. 1996. "Let Them Eat Chances: Probability and Distributive Justice." *Economics and Philosophy* 12: 29–49.
Winterbotham, F. W. 1975. *The Ultra Secret: How the British Broke the German Code*. New York: Dell.

7 }

Can There be Moral Force to Favoring an Identified over a Statistical Life?

Norman Daniels

1. The Identified versus Statistical Lives Problem

People tend to contribute more—and think they have stronger obligations to contribute more—to rescuing an identified life rather than a statistical one. Indeed, they are often disposed to contribute more to rescuing a single identified person than to a greater number of statistical ones. By an "identified life" or "identified victim," I mean Terry Q., lying injured in the passenger seat of the wrecked automobile on the corner of Main Street and Broadway, or Jessica McClure, the child who fell into the Texas well in 1987 and whose family was sent $700,000 in donations for her. We, however, need not know their names and we can accept a very minimal form of identification (Small and Loewenstein 2003). By a "statistical life" or a "statistical victim," I mean the person who, extrapolating from traffic records, will be in a similar, serious car accident tomorrow (and may then be identified), or the children who will fall into similar wells next year if we do not cap them better than we did the well trapping Jessica.

Does this disposition (or perceived obligation) have any normative force? I initially thought there could be no such normative force, but I now believe that a case can be made for ascribing some normative force to the disposition, at least in certain circumstances. Indeed, consequentialist and nonconsequentialist arguments pro and con have convinced me that reasonable people can disagree with each other about this matter, which is my main point in what follows. (Consequentialists claim that we can define what is right in terms of the consequences of our acts or policies, while nonconsequentialists think that additional considerations beyond the consequences determine what is the right thing to do.) This reasonable disagreement about the normative force of the distinction poses a problem for political philosophy: how should policy choices take such disagreement into account?

Throughout this chapter, I have in mind the disposition to give more weight to rescuing one identified victim than to rescuing one statistical victim. If we give more weight to rescuing one identified victim than to rescuing more than one statistical victim, we are clearly giving more weight to one identified victim than to one statistical one. We, however, might give equal weight to rescuing one identified and one statistical victim, but still think it is permissible to aggregate victims, letting the numbers count, contrary to Taurek (1977) and others. I want to separate issues of aggregation from the identified versus statistical victim problem, so I shall not consider the distinct problem of aggregation.

2. What Concerns Are at Work in the Contrast between Identified and Statistical Victims?

Jenni and Loewenstein's seminal study attempts to see which of four possible sources of bias in favor of identified victims is at work in the problem (Jenni and Loewenstein 1997, 237–39). Specifically, they consider four factors that are generally present in all identified versus statistical victim issues: (1) the vividness of the identification; (2) the certainty of the threat to the identified victim and the probabilistic nature of the threat to statistical victims; (3) the proportion of the reference group that can be saved; and (4) the contrast between ex ante and ex post evaluation. Real cases of identified versus statistical victims will include a mix of these factors, perhaps all of them. Finding out whether one or another is the best explanation of responses thus requires describing hypothetical choices that control for the various factors. The inquiry does not presuppose that the bias in favor of identified victims is an error that needs an explanation.

Jenni and Loewenstein expected vividness to be an explanatory factor and mention three factors that convey vividness: the story must be emotional, it must use visual images, and it must be unfolding in "real time" (Rose (2009) suggested this operationalization of the notion of vividness). There is marketing and other research on "vividness" focusing on the importance of concrete examples (Jenni and Loewenstein 1997 cite Nisbett and Ross 1980), also discussed in Deborah Small's chapter. Nevertheless, in their study, vividness was not a causal factor. Jenni and Loewenstein tested the impact of vividness, and the other possible causal mechanisms listed above, by presenting research participants with brief descriptions of different scenarios involving victims. They asked participants to then rate the importance of reducing the risk of harm to these victims, varying the descriptions to fit each of the four potential causal factors.

They were so surprised that vividness did not explain responder's answers that they ran further studies that confirmed they could still detect a bias in favor of identified victims. In later studies, there is evidence that there is an identification effect even where there is no information about the victims (Loewenstein, Small, and Strnad 2006, 32–46). This identification effect works (even when it provides no real information and so is not "vivid") on emotions other than sympathy (Loewenstein, Small, and Strnad 2006, 5ff.) and on other outcomes than rescue. Thus, identified wrongdoers are punished more than unidentified ones even when there is no "vivid" information provided (Small and Loewenstein 2005).

The identified victim is certain to face harm without rescue or treatment, but the danger to statistical victims is probabilistic. We know from other work that people fear a certain loss more than they desire a comparable benefit or gain (Kahneman and Tversky 1979, 2000; Kahneman, Slovic, and Tversky 1982). As a result they may take risks to avoid the loss even when the risks have the same or worse expected payoffs than the certain loss represents. (This behavior is labeled "risk seeking with regard to losses.") This factor, however much supported as a general feature of behavior in other settings, did not explain the identified victim bias. Neither did the ex post/ex ante distinction explain the identified victim problem: that is, the timing of the evaluation of the act, ex post (after the victim appears) or ex ante (before a victim appears) did not seem to be an explanatory factor (Jenni and Loewenstein 1997).

The explanatory factor for which Jenni and Loewenstein find support is another general propensity among people, namely to be more concerned about risks concentrated in a geographical area or population rather than equivalent risks that are spread over a broader group. Since identified victims are 100% of the reference group that can be saved, they stand at one extreme of a continuum, the other end of which consists of statistical victims randomly spread through a broader population. As Jenni and Loewenstein note, the relationship between what people are willing to pay to avoid a risk of death is not a monotonic function of the risk of death—a high baseline risk of death means people will pay disproportionately more to avoid that risk. If an identified victim faces a high risk of death, concern to avoid her loss will lead to willingness to pay an amount that is much greater than what people are willing to pay to save an equivalent number of statistical lives spread over a broader population.

The alternative explanations may have different normative implications. For example, had vividness been explanatory, Jenni and Loewenstein claim that it would be relevant to private decisions about action but not to public policy, for we should not make the amount of media attention, which may enhance vividness, justificatory of public policy (Jenni and Loewenstein 1997, 240). (We might still wonder why it is acceptable for individuals to respond to media-enhanced vividness but not the public.) In contrast, they put the effects of certainty into a moral "gray area," along with the ex ante/ex post distinction and concerns about the reference group and concentrations of risk. In contrast, I later argue that concentration of risk—their favored mechanism—may have some moral relevance. In much of the discussion that follows, however, I keep open the range of mechanisms that may be involved.

3. Consequentialist Arguments Con and Pro

Consequentialist arguments, con and pro, giving some normative force to the identified victim bias differ in the scope of the consequences they take into account. The con arguments generally assume that the policy options—rescuing an identified victim (or victims) versus preventing similar peril to some set of statistical victims—capture all the relevant consequences to be considered. In contrast, the pro arguments often broaden the scope of the consequences by assuming that additional causal mechanisms and effects are at play in addition to the rescue or prevention themselves, such as "externalities" that increase the welfare of the population or motivate them to save more lives. Because of questionable assumptions that reasonable people can nevertheless accept, both sides of the consequentialist argument seem inconclusive.

3.1. CONSEQUENTIALIST OBJECTIONS TO THE BIAS IN FAVOR OF IDENTIFIED VICTIMS

Consider the consequentialist claim that when lives are at risk, we ought to save as many as possible without sacrificing comparable goods. In his seminal discussion, Charles Fried attributes such a "rational" or "maximizing strategy" to "the economist" (Fried 1969, 1417). The economist's maximizing strategy, which takes uncertainty into account (Fried 1969, 1422), requires us to set up a "life-saving budget" aimed at maximizing expected lives saved. Such a "neutral" budget favors the rescue of identified individuals when the calculation of expected payoffs favors them, but in other cases it favors statistical lives. Being "neutral," we value all lives the same, whether they are identified or statistical. Any disposition to favor identified victims would undermine the efficient pursuit of the maximizing goal.

3.2. CONSEQUENTIALIST ARGUMENTS IN FAVOR OF AN IDENTIFIED VICTIM BIAS

Consequentialist arguments in favor of an identified victim bias, in contrast, point to additional causal effects of the choice to rescue or prevent risks. For example, the "symbolic value" argument that Fried attributes to Schelling (1968) and to Calabresi (1965) claims that "we demonstrate the value we place on human life" if we give some preference to rescuing identified victims, whereas failing to do so undermines the symbolic value of human life (Fried 1969, 1425). Fried rejects that argument as "confused, wrong, or morally repugnant" primarily because he thinks it is incompatible with valuing life to save fewer lives. But if we take the argument to be claiming that people care more about saving identified lives and so generate more welfare by doing so, or that the symbolic value of saving identified victims motivates them to save more lives in the long run, then the symbolic value argument anticipates two more explicit consequentialist arguments in favor of an identified victim bias. It might be objected that my argument here rests too much on speculation about the educational effect of symbolically spending more on identified victims. Small, Loewenstein, and Slovic (2007) show that in field experiments involving charitable donations—which admittedly is a private not a public policy context—educating people about the bias toward identified over statistical victims reduces charitable donations to the identified victims without leading to increased giving to statistical victims. This effect is in the same direction as my argument.

One of these more explicit arguments supposes that the benefits of life-saving rescues go beyond the lives saved. If people are greatly troubled by failing to save identified victims and much less troubled by the failure to save statistical victims, then these additional consequences—these "externalities" of the policy choices that also affect the welfare of people—should also be included in the calculation aimed at maximizing the net goodness of our actions or policies. McKie and Richardson articulate this kind of consequentialist argument in favor of the "rule of rescue," namely the belief that we must do whatever is required to rescue people in immediate peril (McKie and Richardson 2003). The rule of rescue is not identical with the identified victim problem we have focused on, but it is at least a first cousin if we suppose that the people in peril are identified victims, that is, that risk is concentrated in these specific individuals. The rule of rescue turns the identified victims bias into a purported rule about what we should do (I ignore the controversy about whether it is really a rule).

The McKie and Richardson argument faces a familiar problem: which prevalent externalities should we count? Unfiltered but prevalent attitudes, like racism or gender bias, may end up justifying morally unacceptable practices. This view seems unacceptable—not all externalities are created equal, we want to object.

Gibbard suggests a way to be more discriminating about the attitudes that we want to count or exclude in our problem. Suppose that we can save more lives of miners if the whole of any given safety budget is put into prevention and easy rescues, with nothing allowed for heroic or very expensive rescues (Gibbard 1986a). Still, we might find it "dehumanizing" in the sense that it "interferes with the direct psychological rewards of human fellowship" (Gibbard 1986a, 101) to simply stand by and do nothing if a more heroic or expensive rescue had a significant chance of saving lives.

Arguably, this concern about dehumanization does not generalize to more problematic attitudes (provided we ignore the fact that some racists or misogynists may not be dehumanized by failures to rescue blacks or women). Gibbard argues that our best policy for maximizing "intrinsic reward" (the worth to a person of leading the life he leads, a notion to which Gibbard [1986b] himself raises some objections) is through a risk-cost-benefit analysis, that is, a "sophisticated intrinsic reward maximization." Such an analysis not only counts lives saved or lost and injuries prevented, but also it counts the "deep psychological effects," like dehumanization, of policies. Gibbard rightly expresses some skepticism about whether dehumanization generally follows policies that ignore the identified victim bias (Gibbard 1986a, 102).

Suppose, however, that turning our backs on less efficient rescues is not fully dehumanizing, but that it still undermines our commitment to rescuing people over time. This supposition is the basis for another consequentialist argument in favor of the identified victim bias, namely, that we can save more lives in the long run by preserving this commitment than we can by ignoring it. This too could be considered a version of the symbolic value argument that Fried rejected, only in this case the additional premise is about motivations to rescue, not welfare benefits that reflect levels of caring about different victims.

A further argument in favor of a bias for identified victims also turns on the additional consequences of a policy choice. Suppose that people encountering identified victims correctly believe they have a duty to aid them, whether they are private citizens confronted with people in peril, or people with professional or contractual obligations to rescue people in peril. Further, these duties need not be grounded in beliefs about the maximization of good effects or the minimization of harmful ones (the duty itself may be nonconsequentialist in origin). Specifically, if rescue squads or hospital emergency rooms are funded so that only "easy rescues" or inexpensive treatments are budgeted for (call this "the strictly rational budget" since it maximizes lives saved per dollar spent), then the personnel in these settings may (correctly) believe they are shirking their moral duties if they have a significant chance of helping people with rescues that are more dangerous or expensive than those contained in the budget. The strictly rational budget then stands in the way of these people carrying out the duties they believe they have. Persuading them that their duty extends only as far as the budget proposes strains credulity.

Like the consequentialist arguments against an identified victim bias, none of these consequentialist arguments supporting such a bias is conclusive. Each rests on questionable empirical premises—claims about the magnitude of the externalities, the likelihood and force of dehumanization, the extinction of a commitment to invest in life-saving, or performance deficits in responders. Nevertheless, reasonable consequentialists may believe some of them and reject the alternative assumption that no other consequences are involved than the rescue of one group or the saving of the other.

4. Nonconsequentialist Arguments Con and Pro

Just as reasonable consequentialists can disagree about whether the identified victim bias has normative force, so too can reasonable nonconsequentialists. Disagreements across the consequentialist/nonconsequentialist divide count as reasonable too, but I shall not discuss that obvious basis for reasonable disagreement here.

4.1. NONCONSEQUENTIALIST OBJECTIONS TO THE IDENTIFIED VICTIM BIAS

Consider the requirement that we treat people with equal respect as a result of their status as persons. An identified victim is worthy of such respect, but so are people who are only referred to as statistical lives—they are no less people worthy of respect just because we can not yet identify them. Variations on this idea insist that we are discriminating against statistical victims in a morally objectionable way if we give in to our psychological responses of increased sympathy or empathy for identified victims. One interpretation of this equal respect view is that we should give identified and statistical victims equal chances at rescue, thus avoiding discrimination.

I note in passing that those who oppose the identified victim bias, whether consequentialists or nonconsequentialists, should provide an error theory to explain why so many people are disposed to the bias and thus "get it wrong." There may be several ways to do so. Echoing Hume, Kagan (1989, 283ff.) states that people form "vivid" or "pale" ideas, respectively representing strong and weak response motivation. Our bias ("blind spot") toward identified victims might be explained in terms of those invoked ideas (Kagan 1989, 288). Kagan's account arguably succeeds only by making a strong empirical claim about the capabilities—and motivations—of typical people to eliminate their blind spots. Otherwise, not being biased toward identified victims is part of an "extremist" morality that is feasible only for a very few unusual people. (Other more empirically based error theories can be found in Kahneman and Tversky 1982, 2000; Kahneman, Slovic, and Tversky 1979; Jenni and Loewenstein 1997, 238; and Greene 2007; but on Greene, see Berker 2009.)

4.2. NONCONSEQUENTIALIST ARGUMENTS IN FAVOR OF AN IDENTIFIED VICTIM BIAS

One way for a nonconsequentialist to defend the idea of equal respect while rejecting the commitment to equal chances is to claim that there is a morally relevant difference between identified and statistical victims. The door is then open to a nonconsequentialist argument in favor of identified victims. To show that the distinction between identified and statistical victims is reasonably viewed as morally relevant, however, we need either a justifiable and general account of moral relevance or a methodology, such as Frances Kamm's appeal to intuitions about "fully equalized cases" and the principles that support them (Kamm 2007, 347–63).

Before turning more generally to the question of morally relevant traits, consider briefly one specific nonconsequentialist argument that being an identified victim is such a trait. Anticipating in part what later came to be called agent-relative prerogatives (Scheffler 1982), Fried considers whether our potential friendships with identified victims can justify devoting more resources to helping them. "Personalists" argue that encounters with identified individuals whose lives are in peril create an opportunity for friendship that justifies additional resources for rescuing them because of the special value of their (potential) friendship, which is missing for statistical victims.

Fried rejects the personalist argument, and for good reason. Many of those statistical lives will turn out to be identified victims for someone or other. We cannot therefore use the potential for friendship to distinguish identified from statistical victims in a general way. Moreover, the relationship between rescuer and identified victim is not really a friendship or kinship that might be thought to confirm special permissions. These points seem fatal to the personalist claim that the potential for friendship marks a morally relevant difference between identified and statistical victims.

Consider now a more plausible nonconsequentialist argument that there is a morally relevant difference between identified and statistical victims, namely the concentration of risk that Jenni and Loewenstein's study suggested was the best explanation of the identified victim bias (Jenni and Loewenstein 1997, 247). Let's suppose they are right about the factor that best explains the bias people have. Could that feature matter morally?

I consider that question by adopting Kamm's general method when she considers whether nearness matters morally (Kamm 2007, 345–59). Three methodological constraints are central to her discussion of nearness: (1) we must consider "fully equalized" cases in examining our intuitions about what matters morally; (2) we must be sensitive to contextual interaction, for features that matter in some contexts may not in others; and (3) intuitions alone cannot determine what matters morally, for we need to support those intuitions with some relevant theoretical considerations. Thus, Kamm rejects Singer's effort to draw conclusions about the moral irrelevance of nearness from very different cases (rescuing someone from a pond at the cost of ruining $500 shoes vs. sending $500 overseas to save a starving child) (Kamm 2007, 247–49 and Singer 1972). The cases differ in many ways (they are not fully equalized as in (1)) and so do not constitute a test of whether it is nearness that matters in them. With regard to (2), nearness might matter if there is a significant cost, but not if the rescue is costless (say, because it involves flipping a switch) (Kamm 2007, 348). With regard to (3), Kamm suggests that the plausibility of leaving room for agent-relative prerogatives in an ethical theory means we may reasonably also think that individuals have some special responsibilities for what happens near them (Kamm 2007, 386ff.).

To see if it might matter morally, consider an equalized case where only the concentration of risk varies.[1] Suppose we have only five tablets of a medicine that can be used either as an effective treatment for a disease (Treatment), provided that all five tablets are given, or that can be given in one-tablet doses to people exposed to the disease, where it acts as an effective vaccination (Vaccination). Without vaccination, one of the five exposed people will contract the disease and then die. That is, each has a 20% chance of contracting the disease and dying once exposed.

Treatment: Alice has the disease. We can give her the whole dose.

Vaccination: Betty, Cathy, Dolly, Ellie, and Fannie have been exposed to Alice. We can vaccinate all of them with one-fifth of the dose we can give Alice.

In both cases, suppose that one and only one expected life is saved (thus avoiding issues about aggregation, but also avoiding standard statistical concerns that there is some chance that more or fewer lives might be saved). In addition, the people at risk in the Vaccination case are identified with regard to who will receive preventive treatment, though we do not know which of them will get the disease if they are not vaccinated. Does the concentration of risk in the Treatment case matter morally? Do we have a greater obligation to treat or vaccinate?

I believe we have a stronger obligation to treat Alice than to vaccinate the five others. (Some others, I know from convenience samples of students and colleagues, do not share my intuitive judgment about this case, a point I return to shortly.) Of course, there is a contextual fact—the scarcity of the medicine. But, given that context, the concentration of risk matters morally.

To see that it does, suppose we modify the Vaccination case so that there are 100 named individuals, friends, classmates, and relatives of Alice, all of whom have been exposed to her. Suppose, as before, that exactly one of them will die if no vaccination is given, and that each has a 1% chance of infection followed by death. Suppose further that we only need give them one one-hundredth of the treatment dose as a vaccination. Again, suppose that exactly one expected life will be saved by vaccinating, just as one expected life is saved by treating. It now seems even less plausible to reduce the one out of 100 chance of contagion and death for each person rather than save the one person already infected. (Ignore the issue of further transmission by supposing that we can quarantine each person at risk successfully in any scenario.)

Some people, however, might dismiss a 1% risk as insignificant, whereas they believe a 20% risk gives rise to a real claim for assistance. What we see

---

[1] I have here deliberately avoided one identified life versus many statistical lives, a constraint that Frick avoids in his contribution to this volume.

from different views about when a risk is insignificant is that the concentration of risk matters at some point or another to the belief that we have some duty to rescue. Disagreement about when different risks should be treated as giving rise to equal claims means we might have to flip coins or, better, flip weighted die to decide (as in some proposals for how to address the "best outcomes/fair chances" problem). Obviously, the issues change if more expected lives are lost by foregoing vaccination of her friends than are gained by favoring treatment of Alice, but that converts our fully equalized cases into an aggregation problem in which more and fewer lives are at stake. Risk concentration may matter morally in breaking ties but not do more—this conclusion would need careful examination that my argument has not addressed. Nevertheless, we might think the moral relevance in this context is similar to the way we consider the concentration of risk in other contexts. For example, Kamm (2010) suggests that we might not hire four workers each of whom has a 25% risk of death from constructing a bridge, but we might build the bridge if we can spread that risk over many more workers, albeit with the same outcome in deaths (one death).

To see that there is an issue of distributive fairness that is at work here, consider that Alice arguably has the stronger claim on assistance: she is worse off than the other five at the point of deliberation about how to use the medicine. She faces certain death if nothing is done or if others get the vaccination, whereas they face "only" a 20% chance of death if nothing is done or if Alice is rescued. Since her claim on assistance is stronger, it would be unfair to her to favor the others, who have weaker claims. If a 20% chance should count equally with a 100% chance of death, then some version of the treatment vs. vaccination case, closer to the one one-hundredth version, should clarify that not all chances give rise to equal claims.

I have claimed that Alice is worse off than each of the five others because she has 100% chance of dying and (by hypothesis) each of them has a 20% chance. If one of those five (Betty) was already doomed to die (say because she had a genetic disposition to convert the exposure into a fatal condition and the others had genetic dispositions to avoid the fatal outcome) then Alice is not worse off than Betty; the vaccination case avoids this outcome if we assume that one and only one of the five will die without vaccination but which one is not determined at the time that treatment or vaccination must be administered. (I thus leave aside the case in which, say, Betty has the genetic disposition to die if she contracts the disease but we do not know who has that condition and so there is epistemic uncertainty about who will die, though only Betty will. Betty here is as badly off as Alice, though we do not know it.)[2]

---

[2] Eyal's contribution to this volume challenges my claim that we can judge someone worse off if the person has worse chances. Frick's contribution to this volume is in agreement with my claim. Frick carries the argument further and addresses the issue where one identified life can be rescued or more than one statistical life is at risk. Otsuka and Hare each also discuss related issues in their chapters.

I earlier noted that there is disagreement at the intuitive level about the strength of our obligations in the original two cases, at least in my convenience samples. If we cannot resolve such disagreement by using our intuitions about hypothetical cases in accordance with methodological constraints (1–2), then we may need to find another way to arrive at a fair choice about what to do, such as accountability for reasonableness (Daniels and Sabin 2008, 43–66). Even if we all agree at the intuitive level that concentration of risk matters morally in some contexts, Kamm's requirement (3) says we need some theory to explain why concentration of risk matters.

Suppose, as Kamm does, that we include room in our ethical view for agent-relative prerogatives. Then, what happens nearby an agent may matter morally, in light of the importance of granting such agent-relative space to them, so that agents may be more accountable for what happens near them (Kamm 2007, ch. 12). Similarly, agents may be more accountable for addressing the concentrated risks (perils) encountered by those people around them than they are for more dispersed ones. We know from various studies that people treat losses as more important than comparable gains. This judgment ends up mattering morally because it affects how people evaluate their projects in life. Being committed to avoiding significant losses (Alice's life) rather than gaining comparable expected benefits (the safety of five people at less risk) thus is compatible with granting people agent-relative prerogatives. These suggestions, Kamm's regarding nearness and mine regarding concentration of risk, are plausible but not overwhelming.

My adaptation of Kamm's treatment of nearness to the case of concentrated risks is not a conclusive defense of the view that the concentration of risks matters morally, in part because of the disagreement about intuitions I noted earlier. I conclude that reasonable people might think it matters morally, even if others reasonably disagree. But if reasonable people can disagree about whether the concentration of risk matters morally, then the nonconsequentialist argument that treating people equally means ruling out the identified life bias also remains inconclusive: it cannot rule out this reason for differential treatment.

5. Reasonable Disagreement and Public Policy

Both consequentialists and nonconsequentialists, I have argued, have reasonable disagreement about whether the disposition to give priority to identified people over statistical ones has moral force. Arguably, these disagreements are reasonable in three ways: proponents give reasons for their view, they seek mutually justifiable conclusions on the basis of these reasons, and, as Rawls and Cohen suggest, their reasons are not limited to those who embrace a comprehensive worldview (Rawls 1995; Cohen 1996). In the face of such disagreements, I have argued elsewhere that (see Daniels and Sabin 1997, 2008) public policy requires a form of procedural justice, specifically, a fair, deliberative process in which conflicting views are considered and rationales are developed for policies that rest on the most acceptable rationales. A fully transparent process that involves appropriate stakeholders who broaden the deliberation about the reasons that should be considered and that is open to revision of decisions in light of new evidence and arguments can enhance the legitimacy of the decisions. It can also produce an outcome that is "defeasibly" fair, in the sense that the outcome of the fair process counts as fair unless it is later shown that there is philosophical agreement on what should count as fair in that case (Daniels 2012). It can thus provide feedback in broader democratic processes that can reconsider both the fairness of the outcome and appropriateness of the process.

My proposal here is that we cannot ignore the persistent disagreement and must subject it to careful deliberation in a process that is admittedly fair. This may seem to be an unacceptable compromise with a view that arguably (in the eyes of some) does not stand up to careful scrutiny, even if it is widely held. But I do not think we can claim legitimacy or fairness solely because a conclusion seems "right" to those more steeped in some forms of ethical argument when many reasonable people hold to an opposite view. This is not a case like the Kahneman/Tversky heuristics that may demonstrably lead to false conclusions under some conditions. There is no conclusive demonstration here about what the right answer is. Therefore, not engaging in an effort to find mutually acceptable grounds for policy would express inadequate respect for the commitments of the majority and would fail to produce ownership or buy-in of the "correct" ethical view. The point is not that democratic might makes right. It does not. Rather, it is that deliberation under conditions that are fair to all parties is the only way to produce a conclusion that people can agree rests on considerations all believe are relevant.

One concluding note of caution about this proposal: No society has a unified budget for addressing these issues and makes policy decisions in one "ministry" that affects all of the relevant contexts. There are many regulatory settings in which we protect statistical lives, and we have quite different contexts in which we make decisions about funding services aimed at identified ones. The hodgepodge of levels of expenditures per life saved may be influenced by the identified life bias, but the bias operates in different contexts and not within any one agency accountable for reconciling them. Perhaps the proposal here, that decision-makers be accountable for the reasonableness of their decisions, can have an effect on the legitimacy and fairness of the outcomes in each context, but producing coherence among outcomes across these many contexts and agencies is unlikely in the absence of some mechanism—regulation—imposing that coherence. Social learning stimulated by accountability for reasonableness will have difficulty finding a foothold on such broken terrain.

Acknowledgment

This chapter is adapted from Daniels 2012.

References

Berker, Selim. 2009. "The Normative Insignificance of Neuroscience." *Philosophy and Public Affairs* 37 (4): 293–329.
Calabresi, Guido. 1965. "The Decision for Accidents: An Approach to Nonfault Allocation Costs." *Harvard Law Review* 4: 713–45.
Cohen, Josh. 1996. "Procedure and Substance in Deliberative Democracy." In *Democracy and Difference: Contesting the Boundaries of the Political*, edited by S. Benhabib, 95–119. Princeton, NJ: Princeton University Press.
Daniels, Norman. 2012. "Reasonable Disagreement about Identified vs. Statistical Victims." *Hastings Center Report* 42 (1): 35–45.
Daniels, Norman, and James E. Sabin. 1997. "Limits to Health Care: Fair Procedures, Democratic Deliberation, and the Legitimacy Problem for Insurers." *Philosophy and Public Affairs* 26 (4): 303–50.
———. 2008. *Setting Limits Fairly: Learning to Share Resources for Health*. 2d ed. New York: Oxford University Press.
Fried, Charles. 1969. "Value of Life." *Harvard Law Review* 82: 1415–37.
Gibbard, Allan. 1986a. "Risk and Value." In *Values at Risk*, edited by D. MacLean, 94–112. Totowa, NJ: Rowman & Allanheld.
———. 1986b. "Interpersonal Comparisons: Preference, Good, and the Intrinsic Reward of Life." In *Foundations of Social Choice Theory: Studies in Rationality and Social Change*, edited by Jon Elster, Aanund Hylland, and Maison des sciences de l'homme, 165–94. New York: Cambridge University Press.
Greene, Joshua. 2007. "Why Are VMPFC Patients More Utilitarian? A Dual-Process Theory of Moral Judgment Explains." *Trends in Cognitive Science* 11: 322–23.
Jenni, Karen E., and George Loewenstein. 1997. "Explaining the 'Identifable Victim.'" *Journal of Risk and Uncertainty* 14 (3): 235–57.
Kagan, Shelly. 1989. *The Limits of Morality*. Oxford: Clarendon Press; New York: Oxford University Press.
Kahneman, Daniel, and Amos Tversky. 1979. "Prospect Theory: An Analysis of Decision under Risk." *Econometrica* 47 (2): 263–91.
———. 2000. *Choices, Values, and Frames*. New York: Russell Sage Foundation.
Kahneman, Daniel, Paul Slovic, and Amos Tversky, eds. 1982. *Judgment under Uncertainty: Heuristics and Biases*. Cambridge: Cambridge University Press.
Kamm, F. M. 2007. *Intricate Ethics: Rights, Responsibilities, and Permissible Harm*. New York: Oxford University Press.
———. 2010. Personal communication to the author, February 28.
Loewenstein, George, Deborah Small, and Jeff Strnad. 2006. "Statistical, Identifiable, and Iconic Victims." In *Behavioral Public Finance*, edited by E. J. McCaffery and J. Slemrod, 32–44. New York: Russell Sage Foundation.

McKie, John, and Jeff Richardson. 2003. "The Rule of Rescue." *Social Science and Medicine* 56: 2407–19.

Nisbett, Richard E., and Lee Ross. 1980. *Human Inference: Strategies and Shortcomings of Social Judgment.* Englewood Cliffs, NJ: Prentice-Hall.

Rawls, John. 1995. *Political Liberalism.* 2d ed. New York: Columbia University Press.

Rose, Susannah. 2009. Personal communication to the author, November 30.

Scheffler, Samuel. 1982. *The Rejection of Consequentialism: A Philosophical Investigation of the Considerations Underlying Rival Moral Conceptions.* Oxford: Oxford University Press.

Schelling, Thomas. 1968. "The Life You Save May Be Your Own." In *Problems in Public Expenditure Analysis: Papers Presented at a Conference of Experts Held Sept. 15–16, 1966*, edited by S. B. Chase, 127–62. Washington, DC: Brookings Institute.

Singer, Peter. 1972. "Famine, Affluence, and Morality." *Philosophy and Public Affairs* 1 (3): 229–43.

Small, Deborah, and George Loewenstein. 2003. "Helping *a* Victim or Helping *the* Victim: Altruism and Identifiability." *Journal of Risk and Uncertainty* 26 (1): 5–16.

———. 2005. "The Devil You Know: The Effects of Identifiability on Punishment." *Journal of Behavioral Decision Making* 18: 311–18.

Small, Deborah, George Loewenstein, and Paul Slovic. 2007. "Sympathy and Callousness: The Impact of Deliberative Thought on Donations to Identifiable and Statistical Victims." *Organizational Behavior and Human Decision Processes* 102: 143–53.

Taurek, John. 1977. "Should the Numbers Count?" *Philosophy and Public Affairs* 6 (4): 293–316.

8 }

Statistical People and Counterfactual Indeterminacy

Caspar Hare

In some cases the morality of action is an interpersonal affair. I am obliged to do something and there is a person to whom I am obliged to do it. I do wrong and there is a person I wrong. Some routine examples: I do wrong, and wrong you, by doing something bad for you, by feeding you contaminated meat. I do wrong, and wrong you, by failing to do something good for you, by ignoring your SOS. I do wrong, and wrong you, by violating your rights, by stealing your stuff. I do wrong, and wrong you, by disrespecting you, by brazenly discounting your opinions.

In other cases, this may not be so. I am obliged to do something and yet there is no person to whom I am obliged to do it. I do wrong without wronging any person. Some routine examples: I do wrong by failing to vote in an uncompetitive election. I do wrong by thinking impure thoughts of nobody in particular. I do wrong by destroying an item of transcendent beauty, never seen. (I say "may not be" because all such examples are controversial. It is tempting to think that the morality of action is by nature interpersonal. Why would a moral consideration give rise to something as weighty as an obligation if it did not have to do with someone's interests, someone's rights, or someone's dignity? So for any putative example of impersonal obligation there is either a hidden victim—perhaps I very mildly wrong each of my fellow citizens by failing to vote, wrong all people of a certain kind by thinking impure thoughts of people like that, wrong all people who might possibly have borne witness to the item of transcendent beauty by destroying it—or no obligation at all.)

And some cases fall curiously in the middle. In these cases a moral obligation may seem, prima facie, to be between one person and another, but it proves to be difficult, on reflection, to put a finger on exactly who that other person is. One case that has received a great deal of attention from philosophers is the "Same Number Non-Identity Case."[1] (In brief: I knowingly, for no good reason, bring an unhealthy child into existence when I could have brought a numerically distinct, healthy child into existence a month later. It may seem, prima facie, as if I have wronged someone, but who exactly have I wronged? The unhealthy child would not have existed if I had acted more responsibly.) I want to talk about a different class of cases, a class of cases that have received less direct attention from philosophers, here. The cases involve actions that seem, prima facie, to bring about great harm or benefit, without greatly harming or benefiting any particular people.

Here is how the chapter will go: In section 2, I will try to give an accurate characterization of some representative cases and of the problem they raise. In sections 3 and 4, I will develop what I take to be the best argument that the lack of great harm or benefit to particular people in these cases matters. In section 5, I will suggest that if it does matter, it does not matter very much. Our moral obligations are not significantly weakened by the absence of a person to whom we are obliged.

2. Framing the Problem: Ought We to Be Biased against Merely Statistical People?

Social scientists, bioethicists, and political theorists have observed that many of us, when we make decisions about whom to aid, feel a greater sense of obligation toward *identified* people than to *merely statistical* people.[2] This attitude is sufficiently robust, widespread, and morally suspect, in their view, to earn the name of a *bias*. They have invoked it to explain why, for example, we are relatively strongly motivated to rescue boys drowning in ponds as we pass them, relatively strongly motivated to send money to benefit small girls who have, in the glare of global media, fallen down wells, but relatively weakly motivated to send money to large charities. The drowning boys and trapped girls are identified. The faceless beneficiaries of the large charities are merely statistical. And they have invoked it to explain why, for example, we are relatively strongly motivated to contribute to programs that aim to cure or manage illness (by distributing antibiotics, for example) but relatively weakly motivated to contribute to programs that aim to prevent illness (by distributing vaccines, for example). The beneficiaries of the former programs are identified. The beneficiaries of the latter programs are merely statistical.

---

[1] Given this name and made famous by Derek Parfit (1976; 1983, ch. 16).
[2] The "identified vs. statistical" terminology goes back at least as far as Thomas Schelling (1968). An influential, systematic discussion of the psychological phenomena was in Jenni and Loewenstein 1997. For an overview of the subsequent discussion, see Daniels 2012.

Suppose the social scientists, bioethicists, and political theorists are right, that we do have this attitude. Is it correct? Do we indeed have a greater obligation to aid an identified person than to aid a merely statistical person? That is the question I want to address here. But it is broad and dirty. It first needs to be rendered slim and clean.

For one thing, talk of "greater" and "lesser" obligations is obscure. How do we measure the "greatness" of an obligation? A less obscure way of framing the question: When you have a choice between benefiting an identified and a merely statistical person, ought you, other things being equal, to benefit the identified person?

For another thing, talk of "identified" and "merely statistical" people is obscure. What is a "merely statistical person"? A person with 1.8 children? A person composed of numbers? There are no such people!

It may be that the relevant distinction has to do with what you, the possible benefactor, know. Maybe you know a great deal about the one person and very little about the other person. Or maybe you know a great deal about the way in which you will benefit the one person and very little about the way in which you will benefit the other person. Or maybe, though you do not know very much about either, you are in a position to know a great deal about the one, but not the other person. Or maybe you know that your doing the one thing will benefit one person, while your doing the other thing has an equivalent expected benefit, though it may benefit nobody—maybe, for example, you take there to be a 1 in 100 chance that it will benefit 100 people, a 99 in 100 chance that it will benefit nobody.

In these cases, there is something subjectively chancy about the process by which you will come to benefit the "merely statistical person" if you choose to do that. The cases are all very important and interesting,[3] but here I want to focus on a different sort of case, in which the process is chancy in a more objective way.

Some vocabulary: Say that a process is *counterfactually open* when, supposing that we initiate it, there is no fact of the matter about what its outcome would have been if we had not initiated it. To be precise: let P be the proposition that we initiate the process, and $O_1, \ldots, O_k$ be exclusive propositions concerning the relevantly different outcomes of the process. The counterfactual

(CF0) If it had been that P, then it would have been that O_1 or O_2 or ... or O_k

is true, but none of the counterfactuals

(CF1) If it had been that P, then it would have been that O_1

---

[3] In case you are interested, I discuss them in my book *The Limits of Kindness* (2013).

(CF2) If it had been that P, then it would have been that O_2

...

(CFk) If it had been that P, then it would have been that O_k

are true.

So, for example, processes governed by indeterministic laws may be counterfactually open. Suppose that, in an optics lab, I have the opportunity to fire a photon through a narrow slit. Suppose I don't do it. Now this counterfactual is true:

(CF3) If I had fired the photon, then it would have deflected left or deflected right.

But neither of these are true:[4]

(CF4) If I had fired the photon, then it would have deflected left

(CF5) If I had fired the photon, then it would have deflected right.

Why? Well, to put the point in the vocabulary of possible worlds, no world in which I fire the photon and it deflects left is relevantly more similar to the actual world than all worlds in which I fire the photon and it deflects right, and vice versa. Why? Because the physical laws that govern the actual world are no more or less violated in a world in which I fire the photon and it deflects left than in a world in which I fire the photon and it deflects right.

And, for another example, processes governed by deterministic laws whose outcomes are sensitive to differences in initiating conditions over which we have no control may be counterfactually open. I have a quarter in my pocket. I did not flip it just now. This counterfactual is true:

(CF6) If I had flipped the coin, then it would have landed heads or tails.

And maybe, if the laws of nature that govern our world are sufficiently deterministic, some counterfactuals with very specific antecedents, like

(CF7) If I had flipped the coin while its center of gravity was between 1.48318 and 1.48319 meters from the floor, applying between 2.899 and

---

[4] I should note that there is some disagreement about how, precisely, to put this point. On one canonic treatment of counterfactuals offered by David Lewis, (CF4) and (CF5) are false. See section 3.4 of Lewis 1973. On another canonic treatment of counterfactuals offered by Bob Stalnaker, (CF4) and (CF5) are neither determinately true nor determinately false. They have indeterminate truth value. See chapter 7 of Stalnaker 1984. I side with Lewis, and I will proceed accordingly. (Briefly: Because it seems to me that a counterfactual claim is analogous to a claim concerning a story—a story whose details are fixed by the antecedent of the counterfactual and the nature of the actual world. But if the story does not specify, e.g., whether the photon deflects left or right, it is just false to say that, according to the story, the photon deflects left.) But nothing of importance for present purposes turns on this.

2.900 Newtons of force to its upper edge at an angle of . . . then it would have landed heads

(CF8) If I had flipped the coin while its center of gravity was between 1.48320 and 1.4321 meters from the floor, applying . . . then it would have landed tails

are true. But neither of these counterfactuals is true:

(CF9) If I had flipped the coin, then it would have landed heads

(CF10) If I had flipped the coin, then it would have landed tails.

No world in which I flip the coin and it lands heads is relevantly more similar to the actual world (in which I do not flip it, remember) than all worlds in which I flip it and it lands tails, and vice versa. The antecedent of counterfactuals (CF9) and (CF10), "If I had flipped the coin," is *underspecified*.[5]

When there is no fact of the matter about precisely what would have happened if a process had been initiated there may, nonetheless, be precise counterfactual conditional probabilities. So, for example, in the coin case this counterfactual is true:

(CF11) If I had flipped the coin, then it might, with probability .5, have landed heads.

Say that a counterfactually open process is *evenly weighted* when, supposing that it is not initiated, for each of the relevantly different outcomes, the counterfactual conditional probability of the process having that outcome, if it had been initiated, is the same. Typical coin-flips are indeed evenly weighted, counterfactually open processes.

Vocabulary settled, here are the cases that I would like to focus on.

Case 1: Rescue One from a Threat, or Chancily Re Robinson, scue Another from a Threat

You know all this and nothing (of any relevance to your decision) more: Some people by the names of Agnes, Belinda, Cyril, Damien, and Edgar are in danger. If you do nothing, then they will all die. If you head north, then you can intervene to prevent Agnes from dying. If you head south, then you can intervene to prevent one of the others from dying— an evenly weighted, counterfactually open process will determine which one (embellish the story as you like). Those are your only options.

Case 2: Rescue One from a Threat, or Rescue Another from a Chancy Threat

You know all this and nothing (of any relevance to your decision) more: Some people by the names of Frederick, George, Harriet, Iris, and

---

[5] I discuss conditional underspecification in more detail in Hare 2011.

Judit are in danger. If you do nothing, then Frederick will die, and one of the others will die—an evenly weighted, counterfactually open process will determine which one (again, embellish the story as you like). If you head north, then you can intervene to prevent Frederick from dying. If you head south, then you can intervene to prevent the counterfactually open process from occurring, and thereby prevent any of George, Harriet, Iris, and Judit from dying. Those are your only options.

Although these cases are artificially simple, they are not otherwise unrealistic. Supposing that, typically, the processes by which we come to benefit particular, distant people through charitable donations are counterfactually open,[6] Case 1 is in one important way analogous to the case where you have a choice between saving a life by diving into a pond and "saving a distant life" by donating to a large charity. If you dive into the pond, then there is no fact of the matter about what, precisely, would have happened if you had instead contributed to the charity—it may be that there are many dead, potential beneficiaries of the charity who might, with small probability, have lived if you had donated, but there is no dead, potential beneficiary of the charity who would have lived if you had donated.[7]

And, supposing that, typically, the processes by which we come to benefit particular people by way of vaccination programs are counterfactually open, Case 2 is in one relevant way analogous to the case where you have a choice between saving a life by way of curing an illness by way of distributing antibiotics, and "saving a life" by way of preventing illness by way of distributing vaccines. If you distribute the vaccines, then there is no fact of the matter about

---

[6] Are they? We have some reason to think so, in spite of the best efforts of charities to persuade us that the well-being of particular individuals is tightly linked to our donations. Our best dynamical models of weather exhibit extreme sensitivity to initial conditions—small differences in earlier states tend to magnify rapidly in later states. Whether it snows in London in January depends on exactly how things are in Santiago in June. If our world is as these models represent it to be, then it may be that, for some pairs of counterfactuals like this,

> (CF7) If you had donated $100 to Oxfam in 2007, then, five years later, distant Belinda would not have died of typhus
> (CF8) If you had donated $100 to Oxfam in 2007, then, five years later, distant Belinda would have died of Typhus

neither is determinately true—because their antecedent, "If you had donated $100 to Oxfam in 2007," is underspecified. Now, we know that our world is not exactly the way that these models represent it to be. Our world is vastly more complex and may be not governed by deterministic laws. But we have no reason to think that the extra complexity and nomological determinism renders counterfactuals like (CF7) and (CF8) determinately true or false.

[7] I should point out that Case 1 is in other important ways disanalogous to the pond vs. charity case. In the former case, if you head north, although there is no fact of the matter about exactly who would have lived if you had headed south, there is a fact of the matter about how many of the affected people would have lived if you had headed south. In the latter case, if you dive into the pond, there is no fact of the matter about how many of the affected people would have lived if you had donated to the charity. Do these further differences matter, morally? This is an interesting question. I am inclined to answer no. I explain why in my book, *The Limits of Kindness*.

what, precisely, would have happened if you had instead distributed the antibiotics—it may be that there are many healthy, vaccinated people who might, with some small probability, have died if you had instead distributed the antibiotics, but there is no healthy, vaccinated person who would have died if you had distributed antibiotics.[8]

So our slimmer, cleaner question is this: Is it the case that, in both Cases 1 and 2, you ought to head north (and thereby save the "identified person") rather than head south (and thereby save the "merely statistical" person)?

3. Appealing to Distributional Equity

One indirect way to approach the question is to think about whether policies that favor heading north in these cases (or desires to head north in these cases, or stable dispositions to head north in these cases . . .) are in some way good to have, and then appeal to a bridge principle: you ought to act in line with the policies (or desires, or dispositions . . .) that are in this way good to have. Another, more direct way to approach the question is to focus on the particular act and its aftermath. Is there something to be said for heading north? I want to pursue this other, more direct approach here.[9]

Norman Daniels (2012) has argued that we can vindicate a bias toward identified people by appealing to distributional fairness. In these sorts of cases you are distributing a kind of good, a *chance of living*, and one consideration that bears on what you ought to do is whether you are distributing this good in a fair, equitable way.

In Case 2, here are the chances of living that Frederick, George, Harriet, Iris, and Judit will have if you head north or south ("chances" of the more objective kind, yielded by the counterfactually open process):

Chances of Living in Case 2

	Frederick	George	Harriet	Iris	Judit
You head north	100%	75%	75%	75%	75%
You head south	0%	100%	100%	100%	100%

---

[8] Again there are other important disanalogies between the cases. In the antibiotics vs. vaccine case, supposing that you distribute the vaccine, there is no fact of the matter about how many people would have lived or died if you had distributed the antibiotic.

[9] I am skeptical of the bridging principles on which the first approach relies. It may be that there are things to be said for policies that, quite generally, favor people who are, in a loose sense, "identified" over people who are in a loose sense "merely statistical." Maybe the effects upon us of our allowing people to die, in the glare of media spotlight, for the sake of people in its shadows, would be chilling. But this has no bearing on what you ought to do.

If you head north then one person will be certain to live, four likely to live. If you head south, then one person will have no chance of living, four will be certain to live. The former distribution of chances is surely more equitable, so, other things being equal, you ought to head north.

Daniels's underlying idea needs a lot of motivating. Why isn't living the relevant good here, not chances of living? If I die, then I am not significantly better off for having had a high chance of living. If I live, then I am not significantly worse off for having had a low chance of living. And why is it not enough for you to equalize your credence of each of them that they will live, thereby distributing subjective chances (relative to your own doxastic state) equitably? Why must you distribute the more objective kind of chances equitably?

Maybe the motivation can be supplied.[10] In any case the idea will not vindicate a general bias toward "identified" people.[11] Here are the chances that Agnes, Belinda, Cyril, Damien, and Edgar will have if you head north or south in Case 1 (again we are talking about chances of the more objective kind, yielded by the counterfactually open process).

Chances of Living in Case 1

	Agnes	Belinda	Cyril	Damien	Edgar
You head north	100%	0%	0%	0%	0%
You head south	0%	25%	25%	25%	25%

If you head north, then one person will be certain to live, and four will have no chance of living. If you head south, then one person will have no chance of living, and four will have some chance of living. The latter distribution is surely more equitable, so Daniels's reasoning would tell in favor of heading south, saving the "merely statistical" person.

4. Appealing to Person-Affecting, Antiaggregationist Principles

In this section I will present an argument to the conclusion to that counterfactual openness matters a great deal, that you ought to be heading north in Cases 1 and 2, saving the "identified" person in both cases. My view, as you will see in the next section, is that the argument fails. But I have found it interesting to think about why that is.

---

[10] See John Broome's (1990–91) efforts to do so.
[11] I should emphasize that it is not clear to me that Daniels wanted to vindicate a bias against merely statistical people in all the cases we are considering. So this is no criticism of him.

Let's begin by looking carefully at the effects that your heading north or south in these cases will have on particular people. Will your decision have good, neutral, or bad effects on people?

In Case 1, if you head south, then your doing so is very bad for Agnes (she is dead, and she would have lived if you had instead headed north), neutral for three people, the losers of the counterfactually open lottery (they are dead, and they would have died in any case, if you had headed south), and very good for one person, the winner of the counterfactually open lottery (that person is alive, and he/she would have died if you had instead headed north). If you head north, on the other hand, then your doing so is very good for Agnes (alive, when she would have been dead). That is straightforward. How is it for, for example, Belinda? That is not so straightforward. Whether it is good or bad for Belinda would seem to depend on whether Belinda would have lived or died if you had headed south. But there is no fact of the matter about whether Belinda would have lived or died if you had headed south! All that can truly be said is that Belinda is dead, and if you had headed south, then Belinda might, with probability .25, have lived.

We have a strategic choice to make here. We could say that in a case like this, when you act and there is no fact of the matter about whether Belinda would have been better off if you had acted differently, there is no fact of the matter about whether your action was bad, neutral, or good for her. Or we could say that it depends on the counterfactual conditional probabilities. If the probability that she would have been better off is very high, if this is true

> (CF12) If you had headed south, then Belinda might, with probability .999, have lived, then your action was very bad for her. But if it is lower, if this is true

> (CF13) If you had headed south, then Belinda might, with probability .5, have lived, then your action was less bad for her. And if it is very low, if this is true

> (CF14) If you had headed south, then Belinda might, with probability .001, have lived, then your action was not very bad at all for her.

I say that, if we ever want to be able to talk about the good and bad effects of actions on particular people in realistic cases, we had better go down the second route.[12] This means that in Case 1, by heading north, rather than doing something very bad for one person, you do something quite bad for each of four people (Belinda, Cyril, Damien, and Edgar).

Now here's a principle with some appeal:

> *A Person-Affecting Antiaggregationist Principle: Distribute Bad Effects.* Given a choice between doing something very good for one person and very bad for one person, and doing something very good for one person,

---

[12] As Alan Hájek (n.d.) has pointed out, even in humdrum, ordinary cases, the most we can hope for is counterfactual conditional probabilities.

quite bad for each of four people, you ought, other things being equal, to do the latter.

Morally speaking, many small bad effects on many people do not add up to one big bad effect on one person. It is better to hurt many people a little than one person a lot.

It follows that you ought to head north in Case 1. You ought to save Agnes, the "identified" person.

Case 2 is a little different. In that case heading north will be very good for Frederick (alive, when he would have died if you had headed south), neutral for three people, the winners of the counterfactually open lottery (alive, when they would have lived in any case if you had headed south), and very bad for one person, the loser of the counterfactually open lottery (dead, when he or she would have lived if you had headed south). Heading south, on the other hand, will be very bad for Frederick (dead, when he would have lived if you had headed north) and merely quite good for each of the four others (each of them is alive and, each of them might, with probability .75, have lived if you had headed north).

Here is another principle, in the same spirit, with some appeal:

> *A Person-Affecting Antiaggregationist Principle: Concentrate Good Effects.* Other things being equal, given a choice between doing something very good for one person and very bad for one person, and doing something quite good for four people and very bad for one person, you ought, other things being equal, to do the former.

Morally speaking, many small good effects on many people do not add up to one big good effect on one person. Equity considerations aside, it is better to benefit one person a lot than many people a little.

It follows that you ought to head north in Case 2. You ought to save Frederick, the "identified" person.

5. How Far Does Person-Affecting Antiaggregationist Reasoning Take Us?

The person-affecting principles, *Distribute Bad Effects* and *Concentrate Good Effects*, tell us that, other things being equal, you ought to save "identified" rather than "merely statistical" people in the cases we have looked at, because some considerations to do with the effects of your actions on people matter, in the sense that they have some bearing on the morality of action. In Case 1, for example, it matters that by heading north you will not do anything very bad for anybody.

But the principles do not tell us how much those considerations matter. How much do they matter? There certainly is something attractive about the idea that they matter a great deal. A confession of which I am not entirely proud: I gave much less money to charity last year than I could have. I think it likely that, if I had given more money, then some distant-from-me person would have been significantly better off than he or she actually is. But I take consolation in the thought that the processes by which we come to benefit particular, distant people through charitable donations are counterfactually open. There is nobody, sick now, who would have been healthy if I had given more money. There is nobody, dead now, who would have been alive if I had given more money. My not giving more money was just very, very slightly bad for each of a vast multitude of people. If I believed otherwise, if I believed that there was someone sick or dead who would have been alive and healthy if I had been a little more generous, then I would feel very much less comfortable in my skin. It would not matter that I would have no way of knowing who this person was. The thought would cause me shame.

But it is one thing to be consoled by a thought, another to be properly consoled by a thought, yet another to be properly moved to act by a thought. Is the consideration "If I do this, then I will not have done anything very bad for anybody" really so morally significant? I am inclined to think not. One way to gauge its significance is to consider a case in which other things are not equal, in which there is something else at stake, something to be said for going the other way. Consider Case 3.

> *Case 3: Rescue One by Way of a Counterfactually Closed Process, or Two by Way of a Counterfactually Open One?*
>
> You know all this and nothing more: A million people are in desperate trouble. You can save one of them by heading north or two of them by heading south. If you head north, then the lucky one will be selected by way of a fair, practically unpredictable, counterfactually closed process (e.g., by way of your computer's "random number generator"—which is governed by an algorithm whose workings you do not know). If you head south, then the lucky two will be selected by way of a fair, practically unpredictable, counterfactually open process. Those are your only options.

In this case, there remains something to be said for your heading north. If you head north, then you will do something only mildly bad for each of 999,999 people—it will be true of each of them that he/she is dead, but might, with probability 2 in 1,000,000, have survived if you had headed south. If you head south, on the other hand, then almost certainly (with probability 999,998 in 1,000,000) you will do something terrible for one person—it will be true of one person that he/she would have survived if you had headed north. But in this case there are also things to be said for your heading south, including this: If you head south then, for each person, your expectation that that person will survive is 2 in 1,000,000. If you head north, on the other hand, then, for each person, your expectation that that person will survive is 1 in 1,000,000. Heading south maximizes, for each person, your expectation that that person will survive.

What should you do? It seems to me that you should head south. I say this because it seems to me that a promising way to approach moral questions is to ask what a benevolent, rational person, someone moved only by wanting the best for each one of us, would do in your position. And a benevolent, rational person would head south. Such a person would not be moved by the consideration: "If I do this, then I will not have done anything very bad for anybody." She cares about people, not about the ways in which her actions affect people.

If this is correct, then, although there may be consolation, after the fact, to be found in the thought that the victims of our apathy were "merely statistical," it does not follow that, before the fact, we have significantly less of an obligation to aid them. Other things being equal, our obligation to aid two "merely statistical" people is stronger than our obligation to aid one "identified" one.

6. Wrapping Up

In sum: Philosophers have a way of bemoaning the fact that we tend to be very much less motivated to act helpfully in cases where our help might loosely be described as "being of merely statistical benefit" than in cases where our help might loosely be described as "benefiting particular, identified people." But there is an argument for thinking that our motivations have tuned in to something morally important. Many of the former cases share an interesting feature. The process that begins with our helping or not, and ends with people being better or worse off, is in some way counterfactually open. Either if we do not help there is no fact of the matter about who would have been better off if we had helped, or if we help there is no fact of the matter about who would have been worse off if we had not helped. So either if we do not help there is nobody for whom our action is very bad, or if we help there is nobody for whom our action is very good. And this feature matters. It is not so bad to fail to help when there is nobody for whom your action is very bad, not so great to help when there is nobody for whom your action is very good.

But let's not get too carried away. It is a further question how much the feature matters. How you answer that question will depend on whether you (as I am inclined to do) look, for moral guidance, to the behavior of someone who cares about people, or to the behavior of someone who cares about the ways in which her actions affect people.

Acknowledgments

Thanks to Steve Darwall, Nir Eyal, Julia Markovits, Agustin Rayo, Steve Yablo, and an anonymous reviewer for helpful discussions and comments. Thanks also to the *Journal of Philosophy* for allowing me to re-present these ideas here.

References

Broome, John. 1990–91. "Fairness." *Proceedings of the Aristotelian Society*, new series, 91: 87–102.
Daniels, Norman. 2012. "Reasonable Disagreement about Identified vs. Statistical Victims." *Hastings Center Report* 42 (1): 35–45.
Hájek, Alan. n.d. "Most Counterfactuals Are False." Available from http://philrsss.anu.edu.au/people-defaults/alanh/papers/MCF.pdf.
Hare, Caspar. 2011. "Obligation and Regret When There Is No Fact of the Matter about What Would Have Happened If You Had Not Done What You Did." *Noûs* 45 (1): 190–206.
———. 2013. *The Limits of Kindness*. New York: Oxford University Press.
Jenni, Karen, and George Loewenstein. 1997. "Explaining the 'Identifiable Victim Effect.'" *Journal of Risk and Uncertainty* 14: 235–57.
Lewis, David. 1973. *Counterfactuals*. Oxford: Blackwell.
Parfit, Derek. 1976. "Rights, Interests and Possible People." In *Moral Problems in Medicine*, edited by Samuel Gorowitz, 369–75. Englewood Cliffs, NJ: Prentice-Hall.
———. 1983. *Reasons and Persons*. New York: Oxford University Press.
Schelling, Thomas. 1968. "The Life You Save May Be Your Own." In *Problems in Public Expenditure Analysis*, edited by Samuel B. Chase Jr., 127–62. Washington, DC: Brookings Institution.
Stalnaker, Robert. 1984. *Inquiry*. Cambridge, MA: MIT Press.

9 }

How (Not) to Argue for the Rule of Rescue
CLAIMS OF INDIVIDUALS VERSUS GROUP SOLIDARITY
Marcel Verweij

1. The Rule of Rescue

The idea of the rule of rescue, as it was coined by Albert Jonsen (1986, 172), is sometimes invoked in discussions about priority setting in public healthcare, especially with respect to offering access to beneficial yet very expensive treatment. Appealing to this rule involves drawing an analogy between cases where persons in dire need can be rescued (the lone sailor lost at sea, trapped miners, or a child fallen down a well) and a patient whose life might be saved or at least extended for a longer time if some expensive treatment is made available. In the first type of case it seems morally inappropriate to suggest that rescue operations are to be abandoned because they are too expensive and that more good can be done by investing resources elsewhere. It might be easier to argue that there is no hope left for a successful rescue—but this suggests that at least all possible means to save the endangered ones have been tried and appear to be vain. In public healthcare, considerations of cost-effectiveness are, however, common, and, partly also for reasons of equality, not unreasonable. Some treatments may be considered highly worthwhile for individual patients—possibly even effective in saving or extending their lives—yet fail to satisfy some accepted thresholds of cost-effectiveness, simply because they are extremely expensive. This especially occurs in the case of uncommon diseases that are incurable, such as some congenital metabolic diseases. For example, patients with lysosomal storage diseases, such as Fabry or Pompe, might benefit from enzyme replacement therapy, but the effect of treatment will stop when the treatment is stopped. The costs of enzyme replacement treatment may amount up to €350,000 per patient per year, which raises questions about whether funding or reimbursement is justified (Schlander and Beck 2009). Whether enzyme treatments are indeed effective in saving or extending the life of patients with these specific diseases is up for debate. For the sake of discussion I will assume that some medical treatments for uncommon diseases are indeed life-saving yet too expensive to be considered within an accepted range of cost-effectiveness.

I take the rule of rescue to be the general statement that saving the lives of some persons who are in need here and now may justify investing much energy and money, even if it is clear that society could prevent many more deaths by investing such resources in prevention. In this way, the rule of rescue involves a particular stance in the problem of identified versus statistical victims. Although the rule of rescue is not always explicitly invoked in practice, societies are often much more prepared to invest money in curative treatment than in prevention (Nord et al. 1995; NICE Citizens Council 2006). This tendency can be easily explained, for example, by pointing out that it is much easier for most of us to sympathize and identify with victims who "have a face" than with unknown "statistical persons" who will die unless preventive measures are taken. Yet such explanation does not justify the rule of rescue; indeed, from a perspective of justice and equality, one should be suspicious toward allocation policies that are based upon feelings of sympathy. Arguably it is easier to sympathize with the nice-looking mother of two children who is in need of care than with the not-so-good-looking and unemployed single patient who has few family or friends to support his claims to treatment—but such differences may well be morally irrelevant. If we are looking for a moral justification for the rule of rescue, appealing to sympathy cannot be enough. This does not imply that sympathy as such is irrelevant. Giving some priority to rescuing persons with whom we sympathize (rather than prioritizing preventive measures that will save only statistical lives) may help to sustain an important moral sentiment, sympathy, that is indispensable in our moral practices. However, where resources are scarce and need to be allocated fairly, just following our sympathies will often be arbitrary and unfair.

Before discussing possible justifications for the rule of rescue, two clarifications are in order. First, the rule of rescue as presented above is about choosing for treatment or prevention, but it is does not necessarily imply that it is about the choice between life-saving treatment of patients with a specific disease X and preventive measures against X. Such a choice might not be very realistic, for that matter, but anyway, the issue at stake is about resource allocation more generally: should investments in life-saving treatment of assignable patients be given priority even if this is much less cost-effective than other measures that prevent fatal disease. For the sake of discussion I will assume a fixed budget of health expenditures, so that accepting the rule of rescue, given its focus on interventions that are less efficient, would imply that more lives are lost (or less health benefits achieved) with the same resources.

Second, focusing on a general justification for the rule of rescue implies that many contextual factors—which could be relevant in specific situations—will be left out of the analysis. For example, zooming in on specific conditions and diseases may reveal particular features that may support funding expensive treatment without appeal to the rule of rescue. If society is in some way responsible for the fact that a patient became severely ill, this might be reason to offer access to treatment even if it is considered not cost-effective. And in the case of patients with severe inborn diseases, who have been ill most of their childhood and adolescence, and have had few opportunities to live a life of their own, offering very beneficial yet expensive treatment may be considered a way of promoting fair equality of opportunity. Such considerations may be central in specific cases, but will not play a role in our general discussion of the rule of rescue.

2. Individualist versus Collectivist Perspectives

It is tempting to understand the debate about the rule of rescue as being about a tension between what we owe to individual persons and what is best from a collectivist perspective. After all, the problem involves conflicting demands of caring for an individual patient in immediate need of treatment and saving more lives, which would reduce the risk within the population at large. Hence, one would expect that individualist normative arguments might support the rule of rescue, whereas collectivist or other utilitarian approaches would point in the opposite direction. Scanlon's contractualism seems to be a good candidate for defending the rule of rescue, because it restricts moral deliberation to claims of individuals and rejects the idea that very strong claims of one individual can be outweighed by impersonal concerns or by combining less strong reasons of many individuals (Scanlon 1998). In this chapter, however, I argue that Scanlon's theory of what we owe to each other—with its specific focus on the strengths of claims of individuals—cannot render support for the rule of rescue. In contrast, a more collectivist approach that aims to promote group-related values does offer some support for favoring rescue.

3. What We Owe to Individual Patients in Need of Live-Saving Treatment

One of the basic ideas in Scanlon's theory of what we owe to each other is that actions should be justifiable to any other person who is motivated to find and endorse moral principles that can be accepted by all. Justification involves making clear that certain action is permitted by a general principle that no one (even those for whom the principle is least attractive) could reasonably reject. In practice such moral deliberation consists of exploring what the implications of different principles are for different persons concerned and weighing the reasons they have for rejecting or accepting such implications. These reasons should be *generic* reasons, that is, personal reasons people have in virtue of their situation and general characteristics: they are based upon what persons in such situations have reason to want—not on an individual's specific preferences or desires (Scanlon 1998). Moral deliberation then involves comparing the strength of reasons individual persons may invoke for rejecting possible principles. A very strong reason of one person P (e.g., *accepting this principle will imply that I will not be saved and hence will die*) cannot be outweighed by combining the much weaker reasons of many other persons $Q_1 \ldots {}_n$ (e.g., *not accepting this principle will be inconvenient for me*). Scanlon thus rejects an aggregative approach in such trade-offs. Yet if the trade-off is between conflicting reasons of comparable strength, the contractualist can make room for the intuition that "the numbers count" (Scanlon 1998; Hirose 2001).

How to evaluate the rule of rescue following a contractualist approach? Arguably, any patient with a rare life-threatening disease whose life depends on access to treatment that is highly expensive has very strong reasons to support the rule of rescue and reject alternative policies that would imply that patients in this position will not survive. How do these reasons weigh against reasons to reject the rule of rescue? The rule of rescue allows implementing life-saving therapies for patients at the cost of more efficient preventive policies, and thus has the implication that other lives are lost. This, however, seems to yield reasons for rejecting the rule of rescue that are comparable in strength to the reasons some patients have to endorse the rule.

Yet whose lives are at stake here? In a way, everyone who might benefit from the preventive strategy has reasons to reject the rule of rescue (Hope 2001). But how strong are their reasons compared to those of a patient for whom the rule of rescue means survival? The problem with prevention is that success mostly consists of bad things not happening, and it may be impossible to know even with hindsight who actually has benefited from a preventive policy. Persons who are vaccinated against several infectious diseases will never know whether they would have otherwise experienced a dangerous infection. Of course, they do benefit in the sense that knowledge about the fact that one is protected can take away worries about getting that specific disease. Everyone participating in a prevention program has a chance to benefit, but few will benefit in the sense of avoiding untimely death. And as far as the harms are counterfactual, there is not a specific person who benefits. The lives saved are statistical, not identifiable.

This raises the question of how contractualism is to take into account the points of view of persons who benefit from a principle that prioritizes efficient life-saving prevention over expensive life-saving therapies. The perspectives can be included ex ante or ex post. If we look at prevention ex ante we include the perspectives of healthy persons who might benefit from prevention. For them, opting for the rule of rescue rather than for the alternative principle implies a somewhat increased risk to their lives. That is a valid reason for rejecting the rule of rescue, but arguably it does not outweigh the conflicting reasons of a patient who has immediate need of expensive life-saving expensive treatment and for whom rejection of the rule of rescue will imply premature death. No healthy person who would benefit from prevention is, at this stage, as badly off as the patient is. Hence, it would be unreasonable to reject the rule of rescue: the alternative principle cannot be justified to patients whose life depends on the rule of rescue.

However, an alternative way to deliberate about the rule of rescue is to look at prevention ex post. This involves including the perspective of persons who (hypothetically) will have profited from life-saving prevention. Their reason for rejecting the rule of rescue is not that it will rob them of a small chance to benefit from prevention; their lives depend on prevention, just as the patients' lives depend on the rule of rescue. For contractualism it does not have to be a problem that we cannot know in advance whose lives will be lost if the preventive measures are not taken. It is sufficient to know the generic reasons these persons would have: what any person would have reason to want given the situation she finds herself in. Now obviously, she will have reason to reject the rule of rescue if it implies that her premature death will not be prevented. This reason is exactly the same as some patients have for endorsing the rule of rescue and rejecting principles that favor prevention. Both the nonidentifiable persons who benefit from prevention and the identifiable patients in need of life-saving treatment can complain that they will die if they do not get what they need. But, as mentioned above, if the reasons for and against rejecting a principle are equally strong, then contractualists may accept that the numbers do count. We have defined the rule of rescue as prioritizing, at least sometimes, life-saving treatment over more cost-effective life-saving prevention. By definition, then, there will be more persons in the hypothetical situation whose life depends on prevention than persons whose lives depend on rescue, and the combined reasons of the former will outweigh the equal yet fewer claims of the latter. Looking at prevention ex post thus results in a reasonable rejection of the rule of rescue.[1]

4. Excluding Ex Post Perspectives?

So in thinking about the rule of rescue, do we need to take into account ex ante or ex post views on prevention or both? Contractualism will support the rule of rescue only if we exclude ex post perspectives. In a way the debate about the rule of rescue can be considered a debate about the relative weight of claims of patients in immediate need and persons who might be saved in the future.

---

[1] Scanlon's rejection of discounting future harms by the likelihood that they will occur suggests that he endorses the ex post perspective. Cf. Scanlon 1998, 209.

Hence, a contractualist argument for the rule of rescue that only takes into account ex ante perspectives would be begging the question. Proponents of the rule of rescue need an additional argument for that choice.

One plausible concern about ex post perspectives is that including them makes contractualist deliberations extremely risk-averse. The argument is analogous to Elisabeth Ashford's (2003) analysis of the demandingness of contractualism, and it points at the fact that many practices and policies are beneficial to almost anyone, but also come with remote risk, more specifically, will cost the lives of some.[2] Air travel and livestock farming are two examples. Many people benefit from being able to fly. Yet some persons will be killed when an aircraft crashes in their city. Many enjoy consuming animal products like meat or cheese; yet some will be victim of an outbreak of epizootic disease such as swine flu. The likelihood that one will be harmed in this way may be extremely remote, but, being in that situation (hence, ex post), one will have very strong reasons to reject principles that allowed the risk in the first place. The complaints of victims against allowing air travel will easily outweigh concerns of all other persons that not being allowed to fly will be burdensome to them. This not only applies equally to livestock farming, but to any practice or activity that comes with a remote risk. Or, as far as certain practices are inevitable, they can only be justified if maximum precautions are taken to reduce the chance of fatal harm.[3] Taking maximum precautions may be burdensome to almost anyone, but those burdens do not outweigh the complaints a victim whose life the precautions aim to protect—unless the precautions themselves are so extensive that they create lethal risks themselves.

Such risk-averse implications of including ex post perspectives seem quite absurd, or at least unreasonable. This judgment of unreasonableness, however, depends on some form of aggregation in which the burdens of precautions for many people outweigh the very remote risk that someone will die if no precautions are taken—and this is exactly the sort of aggregation that Scanlon rejects. Hence, the argument that including ex post perspectives would have unreasonable risk-averse implications does not cohere with contractualism. Contractualists can argue that excessive precautions against remote risk may be unreasonable if every person—for example, as traveler or as consumer—benefits from allowing air traffic or livestock farming. This is because all of them may think that the clear benefits of traveling or consumption of animal products

---

[2] The argument may not apply to cases where we can't know whether someone will be harmed at all. In this discussion however I focus on remote risks that we can reasonably assume will materialise somewhere, someplace.

[3] The example of air travel is more complex, because air travel enables us to save lives as well—arguably many more than the number of people who die on the ground as a result of airplane crashes. Taking ex post perspectives into account, the most reasonable principle would be one that adopted maximum precautions against airplane crashes, including restrictions on using air travel for "frivolous" purposes such as holidays.

clearly outweigh the highly unlikely risk of being severely harmed by air traffic or epizootic disease. Moreover, it would be unreasonable for a person who has always traveled by plane to reject principles allowing air travel by the time he realizes that it will ultimately cost his life. Such intrapersonal comparison and weighing of risks and benefits does not rely on interpersonal aggregation, and indeed Scanlon does endorse it (1998, 237). Yet, as Ashford (2003) argues in her discussion of the demandingness of contractualism, this response will not work if some persons (vegans in the case of livestock farming; poor people in the case of air traffic) cannot benefit from these practices and only can experience the risks, however small, that are imposed on them. Their strong (ex post) complaints against allowing a practice that may cost their lives are not unreasonable and cannot be outweighed by the complaints others would have against prohibiting air travel or livestock farming. Hence, including ex post perspectives would turn contractualist deliberations extremely risk-averse, but contractualism cannot accommodate the most plausible response: that it would require disproportionate and unreasonably demanding precautions.[4]

Let me sum up the argument so far. Contractualism seemed to be a good candidate for defending the rule of rescue, because it restricts moral deliberation to claims of individuals and rejects the idea that very strong reasons of one individual can be outweighed by combining weaker claims of the many. However, the contractualist defense of the rule of rescue only succeeds if it excludes from deliberation the ex post perspectives of persons who stand to gain from alternative principles (viz., favoring prevention). A very plausible argument for restricting deliberation to ex ante perspectives is that this avoids extremely risk-averse implications, but this argument involves considerations that conflict with the basic tenets of contractualism. Hence, unless we find a different argument for excluding ex post perspectives that is also coherent with contractualism, the theory does not appear to offer support for the rule of rescue. To the contrary, as far as contractualism allows aggregation of comparable claims, it will support principles and practices that save more lives rather than less.

For that matter, even if we had convincing reasons for restricting the deliberation to ex ante perspectives, it is still not obvious that this would lead to accepting the rule of rescue for all rescue cases. This would depend on how we reconstruct the problem. If decisions about allocation of resources are made at the time and place where some patients need very expensive life-saving treatment, it will be clear that their actual concerns outweigh those of other persons, who only run a risk of harm. But the policy issue could also be one of

---

[4] Neither can contractualism accommodate the related concern that a good and flourishing society is one where people succeed in striking a reasonable balance between demanding precautions and protection against risk. Contractualist deliberation is about personal reasons of individuals, and collective, impersonal concerns are left out of consideration.

deciding whether, for the upcoming period, a specific budget should be allocated for all persons who will need life-saving treatment in that period. Many of those patients may not yet be identified, and their ex ante concerns will not be more weighty than those of persons who run a risk that will be taken away if prevention is prioritized over rescue. On the other hand, some patients are known: notably those who have been ill already for some time; hence, in this scenario the rule of rescue is applicable to their case, but not to that of persons who will (in the upcoming period) unexpectedly become severely ill and need expensive treatment. In other words: if contractualists decide to allocate a specific budget for expensive life-saving treatment, the budget will only be available for patients who were in need of care during the contractualist deliberation. The timing of decision-making about resource allocation will thus be a decisive factor for answering the question whether a patient will receive expensive life-saving treatment or not. This would be highly arbitrary, if not unfair. How can such a policy be justified to patients whose need for some expensive life-saving treatment arises just after the policy is decided—and who therefore will not get treatment? Apparently contractualism does not offer a clear and convincing justification for the rule of rescue.

5. A Collectivist Argument for the Rule of Rescue

So far we have focused on the strength of reasons of individual persons whose lives depend on the rule of rescue. Instead we might ask what it would mean for us, as a society, to abandon the idea behind the rule of rescue and decide that, as far as human lives are concerned, we should always opt for saving most lives, including those we might save in the future. Think of mine accidents in which miners get trapped deep in a mine, and where no costs are spared to save them. An extreme example is the 2010 Copiapó mining accident: 33 miners got stuck in a Chilean copper and gold mine, 700 meters underground, and all were saved after a 69-day rescue operation. The successful operation cost between $10 million and $20 million, of which, according to the president of Chili, every peso was well spent. But what if not 33 but "only" three were trapped and saved? For our analysis, the question is if in such a case, for moral reasons, the money had been better spent on taking precautions to prevent more mine accidents in the future. A good government cares about current and future suffering, and prudent allocation of resources may imply favoring cost-effective prevention over expensive and uncertain rescue attempts. The Copiapó mining accident is a difficult case for a nuanced ethical analysis given the extensive media coverage that exposed and enlarged any detail of social interest. But also in mine accidents that receive less global public exposure, it is difficult to justify a choice to abandon further rescue operations and divert the money to making all mines and other workplaces safer. The government would be deemed insensitive, harsh, and lacking any compassion. Such concerns will be put forward first and foremost by the trapped miners' families, who probably would be willing to spend whatever they have to rescue their loved ones. Yet their reasons—reasons of love—are personal reasons, and other people cannot be expected to completely share those personal reasons. Fellow citizens can, however, empathize with the fate of the victims and the need of family members to see their loved ones come back alive. In times of disaster, often—certainly not always—people are prepared to share in the burdens of their neighbors or fellow citizens as they perceive the disaster not just as a problem for the victims and their loved ones, but as a disaster for their community at large. Diverting the resources from rescue to prevention might be rational if the sole aim is to save as many lives as possible, but it would in fact negate the importance of the fact that people are standing together, sharing hope and fear, and supporting each other in the face of—and fight against—disaster.

This collective attitude of standing together, sharing burdens, even accepting grave risks in attempts to save or protect some whose lives are endangered, is a form of "solidarity" par excellence. Solidarity is a complex concept (Prainsack and Buyx 2011). Some solidaristic practices involve standing together, sharing costs and risks in such a way that all participants benefit. By joining forces it becomes possible to attain goods that otherwise were not attainable. In such cases, solidarity is just a matter of joint action for a common interest, and hence it is rational for individuals to participate in such joint actions. Cooperative insurance programs are good examples of such *rational solidarity*. In relation to the rule of rescue, a different form of rationality—*constitutive solidarity*—is more relevant (Dawson and Verweij 2012). Constitutive solidarity goes beyond acting for a common interest. As a value it is not universally valid or applicable, but dependent on an existing (or at least emerging) sense of community within a group of people. By seeing solidarity as a reason for acting, hence by sharing in the burdens of some, people attach meaning to their living together. For a value like solidarity to be action guiding, it is essential that a threat to some members of the community be felt as a threat to the community as a whole. Arguably such feelings are evoked much more easily if a threat is real and acute and if it concerns identifiable persons who—together with their loved ones—are indeed considered to belong to the community. Mine accidents where workers are trapped in a mine are paradigm cases—not only because it is easy and horrible to envisage their fate but also because often miners and their families, colleagues, and friends live in a community, city, or region in which identity is strongly linked to the mining industry. Moreover, the disaster and rescue operation will further strengthen this identity, by means of narratives highlighting the perseverance, courage, and trust of both the victims and the rescue team. Note that this appeal to constitutive solidarity goes beyond appealing to the idea that "this could happen to me as well." This latter thought will be shared by all miners, and indeed for them rescue policies would be a matter of rational solidarity as well. The argument in terms of constitutive solidarity implies that the threat to some miners is felt as a threat to the whole community—which could be the village, but also province or country.[5]

From the perspective of the community, solidarity is both instrumentally and intrinsically valuable. It is instrumentally valuable as it engenders social cohesion and hence promotes collective and individual well-being (Lanzi 2001). Solidarity is intrinsically valuable as far as it is constitutive to the community itself and connecting the lives and narratives of individuals in a meaningful way. Policies that insist on cost-effectiveness and accept that "rescue" attempts that are not sufficiently cost-effective should be abandoned, negate the collective dimensions of some rescue operations and the ways such operations signify that victims and their loved ones are not left on their own, but that we as a group are standing with them. Solidarity may render support to the rule of rescue, in the sense that communities in some cases have reason to give special weight to protecting or rescuing threatened community members and hence sharing the concerns of the loved ones of those endangered persons. The value of such concerted actions is not just their outcome in terms of the number of lives saved but also the meaning this joint action and attitude has for the community as such. Moreover, protecting identifiable persons against an immediate threat, and standing with their loved ones resisting the threat, sometimes even involving heroic action or self-sacrifice, may express and promote a sense of community in ways that are unattainable by policies that reduce more abstract risks.

6. Limitations of the Argument

This justification of the rule of rescue is, however, not unlimited. One limitation of the argument is related to its pluralist nature: the argument takes both solidarity and saving lives to be of value; hence it would be unreasonable to invest all available resources in rescuing people here and now and discard any concern about how many more lives can be saved by investing in prevention and precaution. A second limitation of the argument of solidarity is that it requires telling a story about community identity that is not always there. Some risks or situations are more easily conceived of as threatening the

---

[5] Experiencing a threat to the community will be most easy when the threat is real, as in a war or a natural disaster. The argument of solidarity I suggest, however, involves a threat that is in important respects symbolic. The risk that a trapped miner will not survive is perceived as a threat to the larger community—but arguably the community itself will not break down if the miner dies before he can be saved. But if an expensive rescue operation of a trapped miner is abandoned because more lives can be saved by preventive measures—that will be a real threat to the community.

community than others. As explained above, the situation of workers trapped in a mine is a paradigmatic example. The fate of the workers is clearly connected to the identity of the village community, and the identity of the mining village—and of any other mining town—connects to the economic history of the country as a whole. The village community would disintegrate if the miners were just abandoned and preference were given to more cost-effective prevention policies. Mining industries often have an important role in the history and economy of the country that offers meaning to national appeals to solidarity, and national support for rescue attempts. The rhetorics that are used in such support ("a national disaster," "no cost will be spared to save our fellows," "we are all standing together in this rescue operation," etc.) and the perseverance and sacrifice of rescue teams, witnessed by the public at large, may further strengthen shared feelings of solidarity.

But in what other situations is someone's need experienced as a threat to the community at large? More specifically, would this argument for the rule of rescue work in the context of resource allocation in public healthcare? Suppose that several patients with a very rare disease can be saved by giving them lifelong access to extremely expensive treatment. Patient groups and family members may be successful in mobilizing public concern and support for making treatment available, but it is less clear in what sense the disease—or a decision to refrain from offering treatment—is to be understood by the community as a collective evil. Of course, there is no reason for thinking that a strong community could not perceive it as a collective threat or evil. The strength of the solidarity argument, however, depends on the possibilities of telling a story that connects the threat to certain individuals with the identity of the larger community, and such a story is much more obvious in the example of the trapped miners than in the case of severely ill patients. It may be easy for everyone to empathize with the patients and their needs, if only because we all will sooner or later become ill and face death, but that is not sufficient to perceive the threat to those patients as a threat to one's community and oneself. Therefore, applying the rule of rescue to life-saving medical treatment is not intrinsically and instrumentally valuable in a way that is comparable to the mine accident example.

The appeal to solidarity in support of concerted action to rescue some individuals is not only limited in scope, it can also be morally problematic itself. As argued above, solidarity as a moral argument can only be effective if there is already a sense (or emerging sense) of community in place, and if the persons to be rescued are in fact considered as belonging to the group. But is it morally justified to let decisions about saving someone's life depend on collective judgments about whether that person does or does not belong to "us"? Many features may then play a role that, from a moral point of view, are irrelevant: how attractive, popular, or sociable a person is, how long he has been living "here," the influence of his family in the community, and so on.

Such partiality is especially problematic in public policy. Certainly in modern healthcare, where resources are always limited and resource allocation requires a continuous weighing of competing claims, decisions to offer expensive treatment need to be fair and just, and the fact that some persons or their families are more popular or influential than others should not play a role at all.

This is not to say that there is no place for solidarity in healthcare. To the contrary, public healthcare systems that guarantee universal access to basic care can be understood as an institutionalized form of solidarity in which the costs of collective provision are shared by all. Yet if such a system is in place, then the competing claims for finite resources should be dealt with in a just and fair way. In this discussion, a solidarity-inspired rule of rescue does not have a place. The analogy with rescue operations in mine disasters does not succeed, and, moreover, decisions should be based upon considerations of justice and fairness, not solidarity.

7. Conclusion

The rule of rescue holds that special weight should be given to protecting the lives of assignable individuals in need, implying that less weight is given to considerations of cost-effectiveness. This is sometimes invoked as an argument for funding or reimbursing life-saving treatment in public healthcare even if the costs of such treatment are extreme. At first sight one might assume that an individualist approach to ethics—such as Scanlon's contractualism—would offer a promising route to justification of the rule of rescue. In this chapter I have argued that contractualism cannot endorse the rule of rescue, whereas a collectivist approach that appeals to group solidarity would offer support for rescue cases. The argument, however, has its limitations, and though solidarity is of central concern in shaping public healthcare, there are good reasons for not endorsing the rule of rescue as a moral basis for allocating scarce resources in clinical care.

Acknowledgments

This chapter has benefited from a number of discussions with colleagues at King's College, Utrecht University, and the London School of Hygiene and Tropical Medicine. I am particularly grateful for comments by Norman Daniels, Clemens Driessen, and Rutger Claessen, and discussions with Nir Eyal and Angus Dawson. Nir Eyal helped me to articulate the argument in terms of ex ante and ex post perspectives.

References

Ashford, Elizabeth. 2003. "The Demandingness of Scanlon's Contractualism." *Ethics* 113 (2): 273–302.
Dawson, Angus, and Marcel Verwei. 2012. "Solidarity: A Moral Concept in Need of Clarification." *Public Health Ethics* 5 (1): 1–5.
Hirose, Iwao. 2001. "Saving the Greater Number without Combining Claims." *Analysis* 61 (4): 341–42.
Hope, Tony. 2001. "Rationing and Life-Saving Treatments: Should Identifiable Patients Have Higher Priority?" *Journal of Medical Ethics* 27 (3): 179–85.
Jonsen, Albert R. 1986. "3. Bentham in a Box: Technology Assessment and Health Care Allocation." *Law, Medicine and Health Care* 14: 172–74.
Lanzi, Diego. 2011. "Capabilities and Social Cohesion." *Cambridge Journal of Economics* 35: 1087–101.
NICE Citizens Council. 2006. "NICE Citizens Council Report: Rule of Rescue." January. Available from http://www.nice.org.uk/Media/Default/Get-involved/Citizens-Council/Reports/CCReport06RuleOfRescue.pdf.
Nord, Erik, Jeff Richardson, Andrew Street, Helga Kuhse, and Peter Singer. 1995. "Who Cares about Cost? Does Economic Analysis Impose or Reflect Social Values?" *Health Policy* 34 (2): 79–94.
Prainsack, Barbara, and Alena Buyx. 2011. *Solidarity: Reflections on an Emerging Concept in Bioethics*. London: Nuffield Council on Bioethics.
Scanlon, Thomas. 1998. *What We Owe to Each Other*. Cambridge, MA: Belknap Press of Harvard University Press.
Schlander, Michael, and Michael Beck. 2009. "Expensive Drugs for Rare Disorders: To Treat or Not to Treat? The Case of Enzyme Replacement Therapy for Mucopolysaccharidosis VI." *Current Medical Research and Opinion* 25: 1285–93.

10 }

Why Not Empathy?

Michael Slote

This volume contains papers that were given at a conference at Harvard on moral and philosophical issues concerning identified versus statistical victims of our actions. And I hope it will not be considered out of turn if I register a bit of surprise and disappointment at what I heard during the course of the conference. The issue of whether we have more of an obligation to identified victims was discussed again and again by participant lecturers. Obviously. But again and again I saw the discussion proceed as if the only relevant factors to determining whether identified victims have special moral status were considerations of good or bad consequences or of rational/intuitive rules that might be devised and instituted for dealing with such situations. Some of the participant lecturers were skeptical about whether we really can or do have special obligations to identified victims, and, of course, this is how consequentialists are likely to view the matter. They will say that identifiability has no intrinsic claim on our moral concern, and many of those inclined toward consequentialist thinking saw their task as explaining why what seems to be our partiality toward the identified potential victim makes sense in consequentialistic terms. Our preference for such victims can have good individual and social consequences, etc.

But even if emotional consequences have to be taken in and considered as relevant by any consistent and far-seeing consequentialist, that is still to treat such consequences as in the same boat with any other consequences of actions or social/legal practices or institutions. Such an approach does not see emotion or feeling as having any foundational role in our understanding of moral issues, and time and again, during the conference, I wondered at the total lack of consideration for any ideas about how emotion, and/or the empathy that socially transmits emotion from person to person in situations where one person can help another, might be of foundational significance to our conference discussions.

Perhaps I should not have been surprised. This was Harvard, after all, and the Harvard philosophy department contains three of the most prominent rationalist moral philosophers of the present day: Frances Kamm, T. M. Scanlon, and Christine Korsgaard. The emotional or empathic aspects of morality, if they play any sort of foundational role in moral thought and action, are not the sort of thing that ethical/moral rationalism can admit or even, I suppose, seriously consider. So I should not have been surprised at what I heard, and when I gave my own presentation, a presentation, as you will see briefly in what follows, that stressed the role of empathy and emotion in morality, it was greeted with a kind of quizzical perplexity. As far as I can tell, it did not stir anyone in the audience to question their own nonemotional, nonsentimentalist view of morality. No one seemed to think it was helpful to the very real perplexities moral philosophers and others at the conference were raising about our differential treatment and attitudes toward identified versus statistical victims.

Again, I should not have been surprised. Whoever deeply changes his or her mind as a result of a conference? (And who was ever seduced by a book?) All right then, so I should not expect what I am about to say about the emotional/empathic foundations of the moral distinction between identified and statistical victims to change readers' minds. But I have committed myself to giving my arguments again here in these pages, and I will soon be running out of space. What I say will have to be brief and I will have to refer the reader at several points to fuller discussions in other places. But perhaps my Tom Sawyer–like approach here to my own ideas will get people to think again, or for the first time, about why they do not or should not think of empathy and emotion as foundationally relevant to moral questions.

I am a virtue-ethical sentimentalist about morality, and perhaps one reason why such a foundational approach does not get very much attention is the sentimentalists' own fault. There are well-known objections out of rationalism and intuitionism to the idea that sentiment is a sufficient basis for morality, and sentimentalists often have not seen the force of these objections, much less attempted to answer them. One can object to sentimentalism, as Kant did, because sentiment is thought to be insufficiently robust or trustworthy to have anything but an accidental or probabilistic connection to right action. One can object, as Kant again did, that sentimentalism deprives morality of its dignity and even its humanity. One can also object in Kantian terms because sentiment does not appear to be capable of giving us the categorical imperatives that morality seems to involve for us and also does not seem capable of grounding moral norms or standards that have the kind of objective validity and force moral norms appear, on the face of it, to have. All of these—and many others—are good objections, objections that deserve to be answered, and let me say something briefly about them.

My 2010 book *Moral Sentimentalism* considered the issue of the moral reliability of emotion and emotion-based motivation at considerable length, and gave a full account of why this sort of objection does not work. If our empathic concern for others has been trained or educated in ways that sentimentalist moral educators have spelled out in considerable detail, then such full-blown concern can ensure right action—or so I argued. And if one objects that sentiment cannot ensure that we do the deontologically right thing in circumstances where it would have better consequences for people if we acted otherwise, then, again, I sought to show that this greatly underestimates the resources available to a sentimentalist account of morality. I explained at considerable length that the empathic tendencies and factors that underlie moral thought and action can account for our deontological intuitions as well—though for reasons of space I cannot take up this question any further here. (I in fact think, and argued in earlier work, that sentimentalism gives us a more plausible explanation of our deontological tendencies and intuitions than Kantian rationalism has itself provided.)

As for the objection that sentimentalism deprives morality of its human dignity, I think sentimentalism can in fact turn the tables on rationalism and claim that it is the Kantian rationalist who gives morality an unacceptable human status. Bernard Williams's famous "one thought too many" case of the husband who consults morality before deciding whether to save his wife rather than some stranger from drowning helps make this point very readily. Kant thinks there is nothing morally untoward or objectionable about someone who does not care at all about other people, but who helps them and refrains from harming them out of a rational sense of duty or conscientiousness. But this is absurd. There is something morally very criticizable and repugnant about someone who does not care, emotionally and empathically care, about other people, and sentimentalism has an advantage over Kantianism precisely because it can explain these facts, and (neo-)Kantianism cannot.

Finally, my earlier work, following the work of David Wiggins, makes it abundantly clear that sentiment can give us categorical imperatives—based in emotion and not reason. And the book argues at great length, too, that sentimentalism need not be restricted to emotivist, expressivist, projectivist, subjectivist, or response-dependent accounts of the semantics of moral language. Following in part what Kripke said in *Naming and Necessity* about how experiences of red fix the reference of "red object" but are not themselves any part of the subject matter of claims about the redness of physical objects, I sought to show that our empathic reactions to how some people treat others can fix the reference of claims about rightness and wrongness without themselves being described by the moral claims they allow us to ground. I shall say a bit more about this in my brief discussion of how sentimentalism deals with the issue of identified victims, but in any event sentimentalism is as compatible with and as capable of explaining moral objectivity as anything rational intuitionists or Kantians have said on this topic. But now it is time to be more specific.

It is perhaps worth mentioning first that empathy is more sensitive to what is perceptually immediate or what is contemporaneous than to what is only known about or what lies in the future. This is well attested in the psychology literature on empathy, but Hume in the *Treatise of Human Nature* seems already to have been well aware of these facts. Thus, if I see a child drowning right in front of me, my empathy is likely to be aroused more strongly than if I merely hear that there is some child whom I can save via a contribution to Oxfam. Now Peter Singer, a consequentialist who I believe was the first to bring this kind of contrast to our attention, would say that our differing empathic reactions do not settle any issues of morality, and he has in fact argued that it is just as wrong or bad not to send the check to Oxfam as it would be not to save the drowning child. He asks why we should be (morally) partial to the child we see and can identify, and this question would and did occur to many of the discussants in our conference. And Singer has also said that partialism owes us a good foundational explanation of why it is plausible as a moral approach (Singer 1972; also 1999, 308). And I agree with him.

But what I want to say by way of answering Singer is that empathy is not only partial but also a basic ingredient in our moral concepts. Our moral thinking correlates with differences in empathy insofar as we think that what goes more against empathy is also morally worse. And indeed we do think it is morally worse, even morally monstrous, to ignore the drowning child in comparison with not giving to Oxfam. But if the same empathy that makes us partial to the identified potential victim also enters into our basic conceptual understanding of right and wrong, then our judgment that it is worse to ignore the drowning child can be justified and cannot be dismissed on the basis of the kinds of considerations Singer offers. And all of this transposes to the kind of case that was the principal focus of our conference and of the present book.

If miners are trapped underground and we know who they are, we will make efforts to save them that we would not comparably make to save the same or even a greater number of miners in the future by installing safety devices in the same mine where the miners are currently trapped. And that is in great part because they are contemporaneously identified rather than being merely statistical and future. Empathy is more sensitive to what is contemporaneous and definite than to what is future and indefinite, and that helps explain why we are so much more willing and even eager to help the miners trapped underground and why we feel much less impelled to spend a similar amount of money or energy to prevent future mining disasters. Once again, of course, the consequentialist or rational intuitionist may complain that a psychological explanation in terms of empathy or empathic reactions is a far cry from a moral justification of such different attitudes, tendencies, and actions. And, once again, I want to reply that the psychology and the justification come together if empathy is built into moral thought and moral language. So it is high time I said more about how I believe that to be possible.

In *The Anatomy of Values* (1970, 207–27), Charles Fried argued that in the case of the miners trapped underground, we should morally prefer to use money to install safety devices to save future miners if we can thereby save more total miners than we could by rescuing those who are currently trapped underground. And he adds a bizarre touch to his argument by saying that once we have made this moral decision, we should be willing to tell the trapped miners themselves face to face (this is supposed to be compatible with our not being able to easily rescue them) that we have decided not to rescue them because the necessary money that has been accumulated would be better spent by installing safety devices. (We have to also assume that we cannot find additional money, etc.)

Now I find what Fried is saying here quite chilling, and I think most of my readers will too. And this is not surprising. Fried is proposing that we act on a utilitarian calculation rather than respond empathically and (therefore) partially to the situation of the currently trapped miners, and there has always been talk of "cold utilitarian calculations" in the literature of or surrounding ethics. Well, Fried's utilitarian recommendation is certainly chilling, but now I need to say how that supports sentimentalism and partialism regarding identified victims.

I think we feel chilled by Fried and his suggestion because it seems so lacking in empathy, normal and understandable empathy, for the presently trapped miners. Human beings can not only be empathically concerned about others and act to help them on that basis but also can have empathic reactions to the empathy or lack of empathy of other agents. Hume noticed this toward the end of the *Treatise* when he pointed out that we can be (empathically) warmed by the warmth we see someone display in his helpful and benevolent actions toward one of his friends. This is second-order warmth, and in exact parallel there can be second-order chill or coldness as well. If someone is cold-hearted in his actions or attitudes toward (certain) people, I can be chilled in reaction to what I see of those actions and/or attitudes, and that is exactly what is happening, I think, in regard to Fried. But such second-order empathic chill is effectively and deeply a form of disapproval, moral disapproval, and when we are warmed by seeing one friend help another, our second-order empathic warmth at the warmth the friend displays as an agent seems to be a kind of ur-approval of the friend who helps. Hume understood approval and disapproval as empathic reactions of pleasure and pain, but I argued in *Moral Sentimentalism* that it makes more sense to see moral approval and disapproval in terms of warmth and chill reactions. (The idea that disapproval is a kind of anger rather than chill is problematic because anger is typically hot and there is no such thing as hot disapproval. Disapproval, as we normally understand it, is cool or chilly and distant.)

But the sentimentalist then needs to tie approval and disapproval to moral judgment. Now Saul Kripke (1980) has argued that our understanding of redness in objects is based in experiences of red that fix the reference of "red object," and I argued in my book that our second-order empathy-derived experience of warm approval toward agents or their actions can plausibly be said to fix the reference of "morally good." Parallel things were said about second-order empathically chilly disapproval and moral wrongness, and it was shown that this account of moral reference-fixing has the desirable implication of allowing basic moral claims to be both necessary and a priori.

The fact that moral claims of better and worse correlate so well with what we know about what goes less or more against our empathic tendencies supports the idea that empathy enters into our moral concepts and language. (One can question the correlation in certain kinds of cases, and the sentimentalist has then to argue that in those cases, and despite initial appearances, the correlation can most plausibly be said to actually hold. I deal with this issue in my *From Enlightenment to Receptivity: Rethinking Our Values* (2013).) But we can be more specific about how empathy enters into our moral concepts, and what I have just said briefly about second-order empathic reactions and reference-fixing is said with much further argumentation in my earlier work, which does explain this "how" in a pretty detailed way. The account I offer yields the conclusions that moral goodness is identical with having full and fully empathic concern for others and that the wrongness of an action consists in its reflecting or exhibiting a lack of such concern for others. And the explanation also makes it clear how moral judgments can be both categorical and completely objective.

But at this point (and as a referee for this book has pointed out), there is a loose end that needs to be addressed. The above account allows us to see how a contemporary danger can engage empathic concern, but it does not specifically speak of the relevance of empathy to future dangers to miners and others. Surely, the ability to help miners in the future has some moral weight, even if it can be outweighed by considerations of contemporaneity. And this raises the issue of whether future dangers and the like engage with our moral thought by way of empathy rather than, as might appear more likely, by engaging with our reasoning powers and being occasionally outweighed by empathy.

To answer this we need to see how both reason and empathy can enter into the moral equation with respect to what lies in the future. Children cannot think about future dangers because they lack the conceptual equipment for relevant thought or knowledge. And full empathic development occurs against the background of increasing cognitive sophistication. Teens and preteens learn to feel empathic concern for distant groups of people only after they have acquired clear concepts of groups and what can happen to groups. And the same applies to questions of future concern.

A mother who takes her protesting child to the doctor because she has been told that the child will likely be lame, or blind, for life if he is not immediately treated, will presumably empathize with her child's fears, but it is not pure cognition or reason that leads her to take the child to the doctor nonetheless. She is a mother after all, and what life will be like for her child if he is blind or lame can be quite vivid to her, and her empathic repulsion at the thought of such a life for her child can be the impetus toward her decision to take the child to the doctor. She could not imagine that future for her child if she were not cognitively and rationally capable, but I would want to argue that the sheer size of what is at stake—the fact that a future life of lameness dwarfs any present unpleasantness for the child—can overwhelm the empathic force of sheer contemporaneity in such a case. (Similarly, if installing safety devices will save 10 or 20 times more lives than using the same funds, the only funds available, to save the miners now trapped underground, that will make a decision not to save the miners not be a chilling or empathically unacceptable immoral one. The sheer enormity of the difference in lives saved can empathically overcome our empathy with contemporaneity.) So I think empathy need not give way to reason in the sorts of moral cases we have been describing.

However, before I conclude, let me mention an issue to which this chapter ought to be relevant and arguably is relevant, an issue of considerable importance to our Harvard conference and this whole book. In his "Reasonable Disagreement about Identified vs. Statistical Victims" (2012), Norman Daniels mentions the work of Karen Jenni and George Loewenstein concerning the factors that singly or in combination might affect judgments or reactions to cases of identified versus statistical victimhood. And I would like to say just a bit about how empathy relates to some of the factors that have been mentioned.

To begin with, Jenni, Loewenstein, and Daniels himself do not mention empathic sensitivity as one of the variables relevant to our reactions to identified versus statistical victimhood. And I think bringing in empathy could be useful to these discussions. For example, Jenni and Loewenstein consider whether identified versus statistical victim issues can be explained via differences in vividness in the two kinds of cases, and they end up thinking that vividness is not as relevant here as one might initially suppose. Now empathy can increase vividness: if I feel your pain, your pain is likely to be much more vivid to me than if I merely know about your pain. But identified wrongdoers are punished more than unidentified ones even when there is no "vivid" information provided about them, so one might wonder whether empathy can do better than vividness in explaining the just-mentioned difference in reaction. And I think the answer is yes.

Empathy is sensitive to causal connection, and (as I argue in *Moral Sentimentalism*), we empathically flinch more from actively causing someone's death than from merely allowing such a death. But this empathic difference pretty clearly does not depend on vividness: even when one does not know much at all about whom one would be killing (say with a bomb or gun) or allowing to die, the difference in causal immediacy makes a difference to our empathic responses. By the same token, since it is plausible to assume that identification, like naming (see Kripke 1980), involves a causal element, one can hold that where wrongdoers are identified to us, their existence is more causally immediate for us than if they are not thus identified. And in that case empathy may be able to explain some of our differential reactions concerning what is identified and what is statistical in a way that vividness cannot.

Now Jenni and Loewenstein did find that we tend to respond more to risks concentrated in a given geographical area or population than to risks spread over a broader group, but, again, it seems to me that thinking in terms of empathy can help us better understand this phenomenon. Considerations of marginal utility being held equal, the taking of one dollar from each of a thousand bank accounts seems somehow less bad to us (and even to many thieves) than the taking of a thousand dollars from one person's account; and I think this indicates that empathy is sensitive to issues of constitutive compactness versus diffusion just as it is sensitive to issues of causal immediacy versus indirectness. More, much more, would need to be said about this issue and various others that Norman Daniels discusses and refers to in his article. But my point here is that empathy has not been tested as a relevant factor in the area under discussion and, perhaps more importantly, that the earlier arguments of this chapter may give us reason not only to take empathy more seriously as a factor in moral thought and action, but to investigate how helpful it can be to the particular and detailed exploration of the factors relevant to identified versus statistical victimhood. However, that is a discussion that I or we will need to pursue further in some future venue.

References

Daniels, Norman. 2012. "Reasonable Disagreement about Identified vs. Statistical Victims." *Hastings Center Report* 42 (1): 35–45.
Kripke, Saul. 1980. *Naming and Necessity*. Oxford: Blackwell.
Singer, Peter. 1972. "Famine, Affluence, and Morality." *Philosophy and Public Affairs* 1: 229–43.
Singer, Peter. 1999. "A Response [to Critics]." In *Singer and His Critics*, edited by Dale Jamieson, 269–335. Oxford: Blackwell.
Slote, Michael. 2013. *From Enlightenment to Receptivity: Rethinking Our Values*. New York: Oxford University Press.

PART } III

Applications

11 }

Identified versus Statistical Lives in US Civil Litigation
OF STANDING, RIPENESS, AND CLASS ACTIONS
I. Glenn Cohen

Suppose a government official in charge of proposing legislation regulating the coal industry is presented with the following analysis: if you pass an amendment to certain existing environment laws to prohibit the use of certain forms of coal burning nationwide, 10,000 fewer children will develop asthma, although there will be costs to the industry. This is a classic statistical lives case—we do not know which 10,000 children specifically will benefit.

If it is correct that there should be no premium attached to identified versus statistical lives, as some in this book argue, then as a policy matter the government official should be indifferent between this policy and one that prevented the same harm for identified lives; for example, a policy that provided devices that filtered the pollutants involved from coal burning (for example, through home air filters) for 10,000 specific children currently covered by a healthcare program and prevented the development of asthma to the same extent. The official should also prefer this policy over an alternative program that provided the same benefit to 9,999 children whose names and photos the official had on file.

But even if at the policymaking level there should be no favoring of identified lives, that does not mean our litigation system is or should be similarly indifferent. To continue with the above example, suppose that the legislation discussed above had not passed and someone wanted to challenge the existing environmental law (which permits the coal burning) based on the fact that it will result in 10,000 asthmatic children. Who could bring that claim? When could they bring that claim?[1] In the United States, as in most countries, litigation remains an essential

---

[1] I do not intend anything in this discussion to turn on the distinction between omissions and commissions. The two key distinctions are between identified lives and statistical lives and between

tool to change public policy: from the environment to discrimination, some of the most important gains (and losses) in public policy have resulted from litigation. Even the credible threat of a lawsuit can be an important tool for leveraging an opposing party into changing its position. Thus, the availability or lack thereof of a litigation option matters a great deal for achieving major social change.

This chapter examines the way the identified versus statistical lives problem manifests itself in civil litigation in US federal courts. In section 1, I argue that federal courts push for litigants to assert claims on behalf of identified and not statistical victims because of two prerequisites for the justiciability of a controversy—standing and ripeness. In section 2, I discuss a partial solution offered by the procedural rules of civil litigation: the class action device. I argue that the class action allows for the adjudication of harms to statistical victims through the litigation of a representative identified claimant, or a "representative life": a middle concept between identified and statistical lives where an identified life stands in for a much larger number of (as yet) statistical lives.

1. Justiciability, Litigation, and Identified versus Statistical Lives

For the nonexpert reader, let me begin with a brief primer on "justiciability," the set of doctrines governing what claims may or may not be adjudicated by courts. Under Article III of the US Constitution, a claimant bringing an action in federal court must make a series of showings to establish that his or her claim is justiciable—that is, fit for adjudication. Two showings are relevant to this discussion: standing and ripeness. Both of these doctrines (along with "mootness," a third doctrine not relevant here) exist to ensure that federal courts do not issue so-called "advisory opinions": opinions that do not resolve real disputes between litigants (*Westlands Water Dist. Distribution Dist. v. Natural Res. Def. Council, Inc.*, 276 F. Supp. 2d 1046, 1051 (E.D. Cal. 2003); Chemerinksy 1999, 56). The fear is that parties may seek an advisory opinion through sham litigation in which the parties really want the same thing "but contrive a dispute to get the court ruling that both desire" (Driesen 2004, 819), making a mockery of the justice system by having two friendly parties with the same goal posing as adversaries, wasting resources, and potentially leading the court to a result it would not reach if the issues were joined in proper adversarial disputation. The emphasis on identified claimants as a prerequisite for maintaining litigation does not inevitably follow from this opposition to advisory opinions, but, as we shall see, it is instead a function of the two particular doctrines the Supreme Court has employed to operationalize that principle.

---

legislation and litigation. The point is that the rules of justiciability treat litigation on behalf of statistical lives differently than litigation on behalf of identified lives even when legislation does not draw the same distinction. The point can be made with examples pertaining to omissions or commissions.

1.1. STANDING

The Supreme Court has interpreted the justiciability requirement (and the prohibition against advisory opinions) to require a plaintiff to show that he or she has "standing" to bring a court case. One element of the standing requirement that is most relevant for us is that the plaintiff "must have suffered an 'injury in fact'—an invasion of a legally protected interest which is (a) concrete and particularized, and (b) 'actual or imminent, not 'conjectural' or 'hypothetical[']" (*Lujan v. Defenders of Wildlife*, 504 U.S. 555, 560–61 (1992) (citations omitted)).[2]

As part of its injury-in-fact jurisprudence, the Supreme Court has held that an individual bringing a claim must "show he personally has suffered some actual or threatened injury" (*Valley Forge Christian College v. Americans United for Separation of Church and State, Inc.*, 454 U.S. 464, 472 (1982)). In a number of cases, the Supreme Court has held that a plaintiff could not make the requisite showing and, accordingly, has dismissed the lawsuit.

Perhaps the best example of standing doctrine's focus on identified lives is *City of Los Angeles v. Lyons*, 461 U.S. 95 (1983). The African American plaintiff, Adolph Lyons, alleged that he was stopped by the defendant, the Los Angeles Police Department, "for a traffic or vehicle code violation and that although Lyons offered no resistance or threat whatsoever, the officers, without provocation or justification, seized Lyons and applied a 'chokehold' . . . rendering him unconscious and causing damage to his larynx" (*id.* at 97–98). Lyons alleged that the police officers,

> pursuant to the authorization, instruction and encouragement of defendant City of Los Angeles, regularly and routinely apply these choke holds in innumerable situations where they are not threatened . . . , that numerous persons have been injured as the result of the application of the chokeholds, that Lyons and others similarly situated are threatened with irreparable injury in the form of bodily injury and loss of life, and that Lyons justifiably fears that any contact he has with Los Angeles police officers may result in his being choked and strangled to death without provocation, justification or other legal excuse. (*id.* at 98)

Claiming violations of several constitutional amendments, Lyons sought an injunction forbidding use of chokeholds "except in situations where the proposed victim of said control reasonably appears to be threatening the immediate use of deadly force" (*id.*). Thus, the case focused on this forward-looking injunctive relief.

---

[2] The Court has also added two other requirements relating to traceability and redressability, *Lujan*, 504 U.S. at 560–61 (1992), but they are not directly relevant to the discussion in this chapter, so I put these requirements to one side.

While finding that Lyons had standing to recover for damages from the past chokehold applied to him, the Court found he had not established "a real and immediate threat that he would again be stopped for a traffic violation, or for any other offense, by an officer or officers who would illegally choke him into unconsciousness without any provocation or resistance on his part," and thus he lacked standing to seek the injunction (*id.* at 105). Even if it was likely that someone would be chokeheld by the Los Angeles Police Department, Lyons could not demonstrate he would likely be chokeheld again. To put it in our terms, while he was an identified victim of the past chokehold, he was only a statistical victim of the future one. To be sure, though, there are also other things going on in this case, such as the question of the magnitude of risk.

To give one more example, consider *Lujan v. Defenders of Wildlife*, 504 U.S. 555 (1991), which remains perhaps the leading Supreme Court decision on this aspect of standing doctrine. The Defenders of Wildlife organization challenged the government's authority to require under the Endangered Species Act that any action funded by the Departments of Interior and Commerce does not jeopardize the continued existence or habitat of any endangered or threatened species (*id.* at 557–58). Prior administrations had interpreted that mandate to include actions taken abroad, but the then-current administration had interpreted its authority as extending only to actions taken within the United States (*id.* at 558–59). The Defenders of Wildlife sued, seeking an injunction specifying that the new interpretation was erroneous and the older more geographically expansive interpretation of the regulation should be reinstated (*id.* at 559).

The Supreme Court refused to determine the merits of the question, however, because it held that Defenders of Wildlife lacked standing. The Court recognized that "the desire to use or observe an animal species, even for purely esthetic purposes, is undeniably a cognizable interest for purpose of standing," but that "the 'injury in fact' test requires more than an injury to a cognizable interest. It requires that the party seeking review *be himself among* the injured" (*id.* at 563; emphasis added). In order to successfully bring its action, the Court held that plaintiffs "had to submit affidavits or other evidence showing, through specific facts, not only that listed species were in fact being threatened by funded activities abroad, but also that one or more of [the organization's] members would thereby be 'directly' affected apart from their 'special interest in th[e] subject'" (*id.*). The Court found that plaintiffs failed to meet this requirement:

> [Plaintiffs' affidavits] plainly contain no facts . . . showing how damage to the species will produce "imminent" injury to [them]. That [plaintiffs] "had visited" the areas of the projects before the projects commenced proves nothing. As we have said in a related context, "Past exposure to illegal conduct does not in itself show a present case or controversy regarding injunctive relief . . . if unaccompanied by any continuing, present

adverse effects" [*Lyons*, 461 U.S. at 102]. And the affiants' profession of an "inten[t]" to return to the places they had visited before—where they will presumably, this time, be deprived of the opportunity to observe animals of the endangered species—is simply not enough. Such "some day" intentions—without any description of concrete plans, or indeed even any specification of *when* the some day will be—do not support a finding of the "actual or imminent" injury that our cases require. (*Id.* at 564; emphasis in original)

The Court's emphasis on picking out specific members who could show with specific facts the direct effects on their special interests in the damage to the species creates significant difficulties for standing on behalf of statistical lives.

A related doctrine of "third-party standing" might in theory facilitate the bringing of claims on behalf of statistical lives, but in practice is unlikely to help very much. Generally, the Supreme Court has held that "[i]n the ordinary course, a litigant must assert his or her own legal rights and interests, and cannot rest a claim to relief on the legal rights or interests of third parties" (*Powers v. Ohio*, 499 U.S. 400, 409 (1991); Wright and Miller 2012, § 3531.9). Nevertheless, the Court has suggested it will make an exception to this doctrine and allow third parties or organizations to have standing "provided three important criteria are satisfied: The litigant must have suffered an 'injury in fact, thus giving him or her a "sufficiently concrete interest" in the outcome of the issue in dispute; the litigant must have a close relation to the third party; and there must exist some hindrance to the third party's ability to protect his or her own'" (*id.* at 411). The theory behind the general reluctance to recognize third-party standing is similar to that offered for standing doctrine in general: among other things, parties without concrete stakes in the litigation may not be as effective advocates as those who do, and a claim asserted in someone else's name may actually conflict with that person's interests rather than further them (Wright and Miller 2012, § 3531.9).

While the third-party standing doctrine will expand who has standing to bring an action, the existing case law on the doctrine still shades heavily against standing for claims on behalf of statistical rather than identified lives. For instance, although the Supreme Court has allowed doctors or other healthcare professionals to bring claims on behalf of their patients, this kind of third-party standing case does not help very much in asserting the claims of statistical lives. In *Griswold v. Connecticut*, 381 U.S. 479 (1965), the court found that physicians had standing to bring a constitutional challenge to a prohibition on the use of contraception by married couples on behalf of "married people with whom they had a professional relationship." The theory was that the physicians faced liability for aiding and abetting the crime in question, so the "accessory should have standing to assert that the offense which he is charged with assisting is not, or cannot constitutionally be a crime" (*id.* at 481). Similarly, in *Doe v. Bolton*, 410 U.S. 179 (1973), the Court allowed physicians performing abortions to assert the claims of unconstitutionality of the criminal prohibition on behalf of their female patients (*id.* at 188). In these cases, instead of asserting the claims of statistical lives, one identified life (the physician or pharmacist) is standing in for another (her patients).

Cases where the Court has recognized that the loss of income from another party due to the law's operation might confer standing might be more promising as a way of bringing statistical lives into court. For example, in *Craig v. Boren*, 429 U.S. 190 (1976), a beer vendor was granted standing to press the Equal Protection claims of Oklahoma men subject to a higher minimum drinking age than women, on the theory that the restriction would reduce the profits of the beer vendor (*id.* at 194–97). Here the vendors were identified lives but the customers whose equal protection claim they were asserting were largely statistical lives, albeit ones with some known demographic characteristics (age and sex). Still, even here, an identified life with an interest in the litigation must come forward in order for the matter to proceed in court.

In sum, the third-party standing doctrine is not all that capacious (Wright and Miller 2012, § 3531.9; Chemerinsky 1999, 83–89), and one should not be particularly sanguine about the possibility of using it to bring statistical lives into the litigation space.

1.2. RIPENESS

Where standing is about who can bring a claim, ripeness is about when someone who can bring a claim can do so. The ripeness inquiry, which also has its roots in Article III of the Constitution but also in prudential concerns (Wright and Miller 2012, § 3532.1), "'asks whether an injury that has not yet happened is sufficiently likely to happen' to warrant judicial review" (*Gun Owners' Action League, Inc. v. Swift*, 284 F.3d 198 (1st Cir. 2002); quoting Wright and Miller 1984, § 3531.12), or as the Supreme Court once put it, "whether the harm asserted has matured sufficiently to warrant judicial intervention" (*Warth v. Seldin*, 422 U.S. 490, 499 n. 10 (1975)). The roots of the doctrine are again based on motivations of judicial restraint and a desire for concreteness of disputes by invested advocates, with the notion being that adjudication will be more accurate when the facts are more developed and the advocates have real "skin in the game" (Wright and Miller 2012, § 3532.1).

The doctrine has obvious implications for identified versus statistical lives analysis. To return to our example of a coal policy with effects on asthmatic children, when could the action be challenged? When it is passed, though the ultimate negative effect on (thus far unidentified) lives is many years away, or only when that injury becomes more concrete?[3] Policy decisions relating

---

[3] We could imagine different variants of the case: ones where the negative effect is cumulative from day one but does not produce the identified symptoms until it reaches a threshold; ones where the

to consideration of identified versus statistical lives frequently have this kind of temporal feature: a decision will be made at Time 1 whose negative effects will only manifest at a considerably later Time 2, the point at which statistical victims become identified ones. The federal courts' constitutional prohibition against consideration of unripe claims will again make claims by those who are (at the time they would like to challenge the action) statistical victims hard to pursue, because until the envisaged harm is imminent the claim will be held unripe. The combination of this feature of ripeness and the effects of the standing doctrine already discussed may mean that there are private and public actions that will have negative effects on statistical lives for which no one can bring suit at an appropriate time.

In determining whether a case is ripe for review, the courts evaluate "the hardship to the party in withholding court consideration" and "the fitness of the issues for judicial decisions" (*Abbott Labs. v. Gardner*, 387 U.S. 136, 149 (1967)). As the First Circuit Court of Appeals has observed, "these concepts are related but distinct: fitness 'typically involves subsidiary queries concerning finality, definiteness, and the extent to which resolution of the challenge depends upon facts that may not yet be sufficiently developed,' whereas hardship 'typically turns upon whether the challenged action creates a direct and immediate dilemma for the parties'" (*Rhode Island Ass'n of Realtors, Inc. v. Whitehouse*, 199 F.3d 26 (1st Cir. 1999), quoting *Ernst & Young v. Depositors Economic Protection Corp.*, 45 F.3d 530, 535 (1st Cir. 1995)). One can envision these two criteria as a seesaw: the more unfit for resolution the action, the stronger the showing of hardship needed to find ripeness—although the court decisions seem to suggest that both requirements must be met at a baseline level (Chemerinsky 1999, 125). Claims on behalf of statistical lives could be doubly hamstrung by these criteria. First, they might involve events that are not yet final and facts that are undeveloped. Second, the claim of hardship might be harder to make because of the diffuse and probabilistic nature of the harm typically envisioned.

Turning first to the fitness criterion, several Supreme Court cases suggest that some claims on behalf of statistical lives will be unripe for review.

---

exposure does not produce negative effects until it reaches a certain threshold; ones where the exposure does not begin until a certain time lag from the policy decision due to time needed to implement, etc. In this short chapter I cannot parse each of these distinctions more finely, but I think one useful way of conceptualizing the matter is that there are two related but distinct continuums at play: whether the injury is imminent versus far off and whether the victims are identified versus statistical. There can be very imminent harms to statistical victims (e.g., an earthquake has just started and is about to kill someone in the housing collapse even if we do not know whom) and very far-off harms to identified victims (e.g., a model of pacemaker given to 100 persons treated at a particular hospital in a particular week we now know has a defect such that after 15 years it will short-circuit, frying the person's heart). There are complicated issues here relating to whether being at risk itself is a harmed state as opposed to being a probability of being in a harmed state that I will not engage in this short chapter, but are dealt with elsewhere in this book.

The court has repeatedly stressed the need for "concrete" facts, especially when the claim requires balancing competing interests. For example, in *Socialist Labor Party v. Gilligan*, 406 U.S. 583 (1972), the plaintiff sought to challenge, inter alia, the constitutionality of an Ohio election law provision requiring a "loyalty oath," requiring that all political parties file "an affidavit under oath stating in substance that the party is not engaged in an attempt to overthrow the government . . ., and does not carry on a program of sedition or treason as defined by the criminal law" (*id.* at 585). The Court refused to reach the merits of the plaintiffs' claim, noting "that the federal courts do not decide abstract questions posed by parties who lack 'a personal stake in the outcome of the controversy.'" The Court held that "the record [was] extraordinarily skimpy in the sort of proved or admitted facts that would enable us to adjudicate this claim" and that this was unlike "the usual case in which this Court has passed on the validity of similar oath provisions," wherein "the party challenging constitutionality was either unable or unwilling to execute the required oath and, in the circumstances of the particular case, sustained, or faced the immediate prospect of sustaining, some direct injury as a result of the penalty provisions associated with the oath" (*id.* at 586–88). Here by contrast, said the Court, "we know very little more about the operation of the Ohio affidavit procedure as a result of this lawsuit than we would if a prospective plaintiff who had never set foot in Ohio had simply picked this section of the Ohio election laws out of the statute books and filed a complaint in the District Court" (*id.* at 588). Thus, the Court found the claim unripe due to unfitness.

In a similar vein, in *California Bankers Association v. Shultz*, 416 U.S. 21 (1974), a set of bank customers, a banker's association, and an organization suing on behalf of customers sought an injunction blocking several federal agencies from enforcing elements of the Bank Secrecy Act that imposed record keeping and reporting requirements on financial institutions, claiming, inter alia, that they violated plaintiffs' free speech rights (*id.* at 21–22). The Supreme Court found these claims unripe for adjudication, noting that there was no "per se rule that would forbid such disclosure in a situation where the governmental interest would override the associational interest in maintaining such confidentiality," and that "[t]his Court, in the absence of a concrete fact situation in which competing associational and governmental interests can be weighed, is simply not in a position to determine whether an effort to compel disclosure of such records would or would not be barred by" its prior jurisprudence (*id.* at 55–57). Because most of the identified versus statistical lives dilemmas written about by the authors in this book are precisely the kind that involve balancing of competing considerations, these are the types of disputes courts are most likely to find to be unripe due to lack of fitness for adjudication.

The cases finding unripeness based primarily on the hardship criterion are more varied in their fact patterns. The Supreme Court has been more likely to find ripeness when the challenging party is forced to choose between forgoing allegedly lawful behavior or facing the risk of prosecution with substantial consequences (Chemerinsky 1999, 118). Chemerinsky contrasts two Supreme Court holdings on this score (Chemerinsky 1999, 118–19): In *Abbott Laboratories v. Gardner*, 387 U.S. 136, 152–53 (1967), the Court allowed a drug company to challenge an FDA regulation before any enforcement because otherwise the company would have to "change all their labels, advertisements, and promotional materials" and "destroy stocks of printed matter," or refuse to do so and "risk serious criminal and civil penalties for the unlawful distribution of 'misbranded' drugs." By contrast, in *Toilet Goods Association, Inc. v. Gardner*, 387 U.S. 158 (1967), all that was required of the complaining plaintiff was to permit "reasonable inspection of a 'factory, warehouse, establishment, or vehicle and all pertinent equipment, finished and unfinished materials; containers, and labeling therein,'" and the Court noted "no irremediable adverse consequences flow from requiring a later challenge to this regulation by a manufacturer who refuses to allow this type of inspection" because "a refusal to admit an inspector here would at most lead only to a suspension of certification services to the particular party, a determination that can then be promptly challenged through an administrative procedure, which in turn is reviewable by a court" (*id*. at 164–65).

The contexts of these decisions are different from the typical statistical versus identified lives policy dilemmas, so it is hard to say much that is generalizable as to the hardship issue. On the one hand, many of the policy dilemmas involving statistical lives share with cases like *Abbott* an irreversibility element because the money has already been spent or it is too late to ramp up investment at the time that identified lives are present. On the other hand, in many of these cases, the injuries will be probabilistic and speculative, which the Supreme Court has held to disfavor ripeness. For example, *Reno v. Catholic Social Services*, 509 U.S. 43 (1993), involved a challenge to INS interpretations of a federal statute providing that undocumented aliens who wished to reside permanently had to apply first for temporary resident status by establishing, among other things, that they had resided continuously, and had been physically present continuously for specified periods, in the United States (*id*. at 43). When a "class of plaintiffs, Catholic Social Services, challenged" the regulation through class actions, the Court found their challenge unripe for review because "it was entirely speculative whether any members of the class would be denied legalization because of the regulations"; the Court said the "case may be ripe for review if the immigrants took the additional step of apply[ing] for legalization," but not before (Chemerinsky 1999, 124). Technically speaking, the Court's problem in this case was that it was speculative that anyone would be adversely affected by the regulation in question (i.e., not being convinced of the probability of injury to anyone), rather than the Court being convinced that someone would be harmed but not knowing if the plaintiffs were one of that class (i.e., not being convinced of the probability that a particular party bringing the claim would be among those injured), a true statistical versus identified lives problem. Still, the tendency to view speculative injuries as unripe exacerbates the tendency to disfavor statistical lives in litigation, because many claims on behalf of statistical lives will also be speculative and probabilistic.

This brief tour of the Supreme Court's justiciability case law relating to standing (particularly injury-in-fact) and ripeness demonstrates that even if policymakers stop favoring identified over statistical lives, when it comes to policy decisions made through litigation, the justiciability doctrines that derive from the Constitution and prudential concerns strongly favor claims made on behalf of identified lives and make it much more difficult to litigate on behalf of statistical lives. Additionally, although this federal case law is not binding in US state court systems, which may have their own standing rules and ripeness rules (Hall 2011, 1270–72; Linde 2005, 1275), many of these state courts have adopted standing rules that are similarly restrictive and a problem for statistical lives claims (Doggett 2008, 855–63). Therefore, plaintiffs will face similar difficulties in state courts.

2. Class Actions and the "Representative Victim" as a Partial Solution

What the litigation system takes from statistical victims, on the one hand, however, it partially gives back via the class action device. A class action is a lawsuit in which a large group of plaintiffs collectively bring a suit in court (or, less commonly, the suit is brought against a large number of defendants). Although collective actions date to the year 1199 in the court of the archbishop of Canterbury, the modern class action had its debut in the promulgation of the Federal Rules of Civil Procedure in 1938, with earlier precursors in equity practice (Yeazell 1997, 687–88; Wright and Miller 2012, § 1752).

In the class action, the ideal of an actual day in court that is at the center of American litigation values is replaced with a "representative" day in court, where we hold that the absent class member's due process rights are fulfilled by way of the class representatives' day in court. For this substitution to be acceptable, the federal court system requires meeting several prerequisites to balance the advantages of aggregate litigation (especially for small claims plaintiffs who otherwise would not be inclined or able to vindicate suits) against the threat to due process where someone else represents an individual and whose representation will preclude the individual from bringing his or her own future action.

Stated briefly, to bring a class action the plaintiff must show that the following requirements (called the requirements for "certification") are met: the boundaries of the class are identifiable and definite; the class representative is a member of the class; the class is numerous such that other forms of litigation is impracticable; there "are questions of law or fact common to the class"; "the claims or defenses of the representative parties are typical of the claims or defenses of the class"; and "the representative parties will fairly and adequately protect the interests of the class" (Fed. R. Civ. P. 23). Plaintiffs also must fit their class actions into one of several standard types, and for actions seeking predominantly money damages they must make a further showing that "questions of law or fact common to class members predominate over any questions affecting only individual members, and that a class action is superior to other available methods for fairly and efficiently adjudicating the controversy" (*id.*).

One way of understanding the class action is that it splits the difference between identified and statistical lives through the notion of a "representative life" (my own term). Thus, in describing the class of people whose claims will be litigated, one need not limit oneself to a description of people who are *presently* identifiable; statistical lives may be class members so long as the class representative is an identifiable life.

For example, consider a class action certified in Delaware for white firefighters who alleged they were unlawfully discriminated against for promotion due to their race (*Wilmington Firefighters Local 1590 v. City of Wilmington*, 109 F.R.D. 89 (D. Del 1985)). The class proposed and certified was "All present or future uniformed employees of the City of Wilmington Fire Department who took the 1984 promotional exam or, who are eligible for future promotional exams, whose position on the 1984 promotion list or on any future promotion lists was or may in the future be affected by the City of Wilmington's interpretation of its obligations . . . to require alteration of the scoring system of promotional examinations for the purpose of increasing the number or percentage of minority promotions" (*id.* at 91). The class representative, Dennis M. Kirlin, a white firefighter who alleged he was unlawfully denied promotion, was allowed to serve as a stand-in for some identifiable lives—others who were already unlawfully denied promotion—as well as some true statistical lives—those who "may in the future be affected." Thus, in class actions, a representative life may get statistical lives into court and have their claims litigated.

The class action is only a partial salve for federal courts' bias against statistical lives, for two reasons. First, there must be an identified life to serve as the representative life bringing a claim on behalf of the statistical life. That identified life must meet the requirements of standing and ripeness in his or her claim, which as we have seen may pose some difficulties. Second, the prerequisites for bringing a class action in the federal system and achieving certification are not easy, and the Supreme Court has made policing of the prerequisites more vigorous in recent cases. In particular, *Wal-Mart Stores, Inc. v. Dukes*, 131 S. Ct. 2541 (2011), increased the demands of the commonality prerequisite for class certification (requiring "questions of law or fact common to the class") such that the courts will now require much more similarity in claims between the representative plaintiff and the absent class members. Although it may still be too early to tell the full fallout of this decision, the more difficult it is to bring a case in the form of a class action, the less valuable class actions are as a way of partially countering the federal courts' bias against claims on behalf of statistical lives. To be sure, even if class actions were easy to bring, and even if we were to relax the ripeness and standing doctrines, litigation, as a way of achieving public policy objectives, would not be perfectly indifferent between identified and statistical lives, for many reasons. Chief among them is that litigation is not free, and it is much harder to finance a court challenge when the winners and losers are only statistical, not identified.

3. Conclusion

Much of the literature on the identified versus statistical lives issue focuses on "policy decisions" generally. Yet while many policy decisions are made by the legislative and executive branches of government, litigation also represents an important form of policymaking, both in announcing new rules, shaping existing legislative interpretations, and enforcing existing legislative rules, as well as regulating conduct between private parties. Considering litigation in the US federal courts, there is a significant bias in favor of identified lives. I focus on two of the biggest sources of this bias stemming from the justiciability doctrines of standing and ripeness. At the same time, the class action device offers an intermediate concept, a "representative life," wherein an identified life is allowed to stand in for a statistical life. While the class action device has significant procedural limitations of its own, it allows one way for statistical lives to make their way back into litigation, although for the reasons I discuss, it is only a partial salve. The concept of a representative life may also be helpful as a way of getting nonjudicial decision-makers to take seriously the fates of statistical lives, by framing for them the idea that there are "thousands of people just like Jim whom this decision will affect," where Jim is a fully fleshed-out identified life that can serve the function of a representative life.

Acknowledgments

I thank Norman Daniels, Nir Eyal, Nicholson Price, and Jim Greiner for comments on earlier drafts. Ashwin Phatak provided excellent research assistance, for which I thank him. This work was funded by support from the Greenwall Foundation and the Radcliffe Institute for Advance Studies at Harvard University.

References

Chemerinsky, Erwin. 1999. *Federal Jurisdiction*. 3d ed. Gaithersburg, MD: Aspen Law & Business.

Doggett, James W. 2008. "'Trickle Down' Constitutional Interpretation: Should Federal Limits on Legislative Conferral of Standing Be Imported into State Constitutional Law?" *Columbia Law Review* 108: 839–81.

Driesen, David M. 2004. "Standing for Nothing: The Paradox of Demanding Concrete Context for Formalist Adjudication." *Cornell Law Review* 89: 808–91.

Hall, Matthew I. 2011. "Asymmetrical Jurisdiction." *UCLA Law Review* 58: 1257–302.

Linde, Hans A. 2005. "The State and the Federal Courts in Governance: Vive La Différence!" *William and Mary Law Review* 46: 1273–88.

Yeazell, Stephen C. 1997. "The Past and Future of Defendant and Settlement Classes in Collective Litigation." *Arizona Law Review* 39: 687–704.

Wright, Charles Alan, Arthur R. Miller, and Edward H. Cooper. 1984. *Federal Practice and Procedure* 13A. 2d ed. St. Paul, MN: West.

———. 2012. *Federal Practice & Procedure* 13A. 3d ed. St. Paul, MN: West.

12 }

Statistical Lives in Environmental Law

Lisa Heinzerling

The life of environmental law is the statistical life. It is barely an exaggeration to say there are no identified lives in environmental law. In fact, as it relates to human health, environmental law is arguably defined by reference to the protection of statistical, not identified, lives. Environmental law is forward-looking and preventative, not backward-looking and compensatory. This future-oriented framework turns our attention to coming probabilities, spread across human populations, rather than to past events, visited upon individuals, and thus it fixes our gaze on statistical rather than identified lives. In addition, environmental risks themselves are generalized and probabilistic, not individualized and certain. The health conditions associated with pollution—cancers of many kinds, heart attacks, asthma, bronchitis, neurological deficits, reproductive abnormalities, and more—are common even without pollution. Both before and after the fact, it is difficult if not impossible to say exactly which sufferers of these conditions are the victims of pollution.

Indeed, when victims are, unarguably, identified, we sometimes categorize the cause of their harm as something other than "environmental," even if, in the abstract, it is hard to see why it is not an environmental problem. When eleven workers died on the Deepwater Horizon oil rig in the Gulf of Mexico, their deaths were attributed to a workplace safety problem rather than an environmental problem, even though the very same problem also led to the worst oil spill in US history. The association of environmental law with statistical rather than identified lives is so strong that we often seem disinclined to think of identified victims as environmental casualties.

Given the general preference for protecting identified over statistical lives, as discussed and debated in other chapters in this book, and given environmental law's focus on the latter rather than the former, one might expect environmental law to offer relatively weak protections for human health. But just the opposite is true. The major US environmental laws, at least as written, offer exceedingly strong protections for human health. Environmental legal standards based explicitly on protection of human health tend to be very strict, almost unyieldingly so. Many examples exist; I will rest with citing a handful.

In the United States, the predominant federal law regulating air pollution is the Clean Air Act, which is implemented by the predominant federal environmental agency, the Environmental Protection Agency (EPA). The primary National Ambient Air Quality Standards of the Clean Air Act—the centerpiece of that statute and of its many regulatory offshoots—must be based exclusively on scientific evidence of the effects of air pollution on human health (*Whitman v. American Trucking Associations*, 531 U.S. 457 (2001)). Costs are legally irrelevant; technological feasibility is irrelevant; hardships posed to the implementing states are irrelevant. These standards must, moreover, protect all populations with an adequate margin of safety: the old as well as the young, the sick as well as the healthy, urbanites as well as rural populations (*Lead Industries Association v. EPA*, 647 F.2d 1130, 1153 (D.C. Cir. 1980)). All of the lives protected by this complex and expensive program have been statistical lives; no rulemaking in the forty-plus-year history of this program has ever identified a single individual victim of air pollution. The statistical life, in other words, is the sole, well-protected beneficiary of our signature national air pollution program.

Another important program of the Clean Air Act, regulating toxic air pollutants, also requires strong protections for statistical lives. Sources of these pollutants must use the very best control technology to reduce the pollutants—even if, in the case of new sources, only one other facility in the country uses that control technology (42 U.S.C. 7412(d)(3)). Beyond requiring the very best pollution control technology, the act also requires EPA to set even stricter limits if unacceptable residual risks to humans remain after the best technology has been installed (42 U.S.C. 7412(f)(2)(A)). When the risks to human health include cancer, unacceptable residual risk is defined by reference to a benchmark of an individual risk of greater than 1 in 1,000,000 (42 U.S.C. 7412(f)(2)(A)). Although, as we will see, this benchmark in practice allows great variability (and many deaths), as written it seems to gesture toward a world in which people are protected from all but the tiniest risks posed by toxic air pollutants. Here, too, the statistical life appears to be generously protected.

The same degree of protection is offered to children by the federal law regulating pesticides. Under the Food Quality Protection Act, EPA is to assure children a "reasonable certainty of no harm" due to pesticides (21 U.S.C. 346a(b)(2)(c)(ii)(I)). This level of protection is understood to refer to a risk of less than 1 in 1,000,000 (H.R. Rep. No. 104-669, pt. 2 at 41 (1996)). Compare this risk to the benchmark risk aimed for under the Occupational Safety and Health Act (1 in 1,000) (Adler 2005, 1170), and it is easy to see how relatively solicitous environmental law is toward the statistical life.

Environmental law, in short, appears to take the statistical life very seriously. The statistical life is really the only life in environmental law, and it is supposed to be protected, sometimes at all costs. In environmental law as written, therefore, we see a possible exception to the usual divide between protections afforded statistical lives and those given to identified lives; here, perhaps, statistical lives are treated with the same care as identified lives.

In reality, however, environmental law does not live up to its protective promise. This is not to say that environmental laws have failed. On the contrary, they have protected untold numbers of people from pollution-related illness and death. Nevertheless, the law in operation allows many people to die. Indeed, often enough, the government looks human lives in the eye (so to speak) and affirmatively—consciously, deliberately, sometimes even sanctimoniously—decides not to protect them. This, in a context in which the lives are endangered by the preventable actions of other people. It is as if Baby Jessica did not fall into well, but was about to be pushed into a well, and we stood by and did nothing, consciously deciding not to help her. And then congratulated ourselves for our forbearance.

When the government does this—when it consciously decides not to protect people from being killed by the polluting activities of other people—it explains itself in terms that trade on the concept of statistical life. In this way, despite the formal importance of the statistical life in environmental law, the statistical life remains a second-class citizen in this domain as well as others.

In defending decisions to allow people to die, in terms that, implicitly or explicitly, take advantage of the generally lower status of the statistical life, the government has used at least three different approaches. The first is to ignore lives altogether and focus only on costs; the second is to downplay lives and focus on individual risks; and the third is to balance lives against the costs of protecting them and to find that the lives do not outweigh the costs. Under each approach, the effect is to move us away from solicitude and toward nonchalance in our relationship to the statistical life.

One rationale for failing to protect against deaths caused by pollution focuses solely on economic costs. Here, the government decides that the costs of life-saving action are just too great, period. Focusing on only the costs of protection effectively ignores the lives lost without that protection. Perhaps the most prominent recent example of this kind of choice is President Obama's decision to direct EPA Administrator Lisa Jackson to withdraw an air quality standard for ozone, which she had sent to the White House for review (Administration of Barack Obama 2011). EPA estimated that its standard would likely save thousands of lives per year (EPA 2011, 26, table S2.1). The standard was to be set under the provisions of the Clean Air Act that I mentioned previously, forbidding consideration of economic costs and other factors related to feasibility. Even so, the president explained his decision by reference to the challenging economic times and the desire to avoid "regulatory burdens and regulatory uncertainty" (Administration of Barack Obama 2011). The president did not explain why these factors outweighed the lives to be saved by the rule; indeed, neither he nor his surrogates mentioned these lives at all in defending the president's choice. In fact, when representatives of public health and environmental groups raised the issue in a meeting with William Daley, then the White House chief of staff, Mr. Daley asked: "What are the health impacts of unemployment?" (Broder 2011).

If the lives to be saved by the ozone standard had been identified lives—if several thousand people had been trapped in a coal mine and the president had to decide whether to rescue them—it is hard to believe the decision would have been framed as it was (solely in terms of costs) or even come out as it did (against the lives). Compare the president's response to the possibility of a massacre at the hands of Muammar Gaddafi's forces in Libya: defending his decision to join other countries in using air strikes to prevent these deaths, President Obama referred to the alternative of inaction and said simply, "That's not who we are" (Lewis 2012).

Of course, there are many differences between Libya and ozone. But the number of lives at stake in both cases was large, and yet in one instance the president talked only about the costs, and not the lives, and in the other he spoke only of the lives, and not the costs. It is not implausible to think that the statistical nature of the lives at stake in the ozone matter made it possible simply to erase them from the decision-making ledger.

Another defense of decisions to allow pollution-related deaths turns the same individual risk threshold cited earlier as evidence of strong protection of the statistical life into a shield against what the government regards as undue protection. In setting standards for air toxins, after the best control technologies have been installed, EPA decides whether to require further controls by determining how much risk is acceptable. If pollution is below the level of acceptable risk, then EPA does not require further protection. The agency has concluded that the most pertinent question here is not how many human lives it is acceptable to sacrifice, but how large a risk is acceptable to bear. In recent rules on air toxins, for example, EPA determined that a risk of 100 in 1,000,000 was acceptable (EPA 2009). Since pollution control technologies had already reduced risks below this level, EPA concluded that its work was done—even if human lives were lost. The risk was acceptable; therefore the loss in life was acceptable, too.

The transfer of focus from lives to risk would not be possible with identified lives. Identified lives are not described in terms of individual risks posed to a population of people; that is part of the definition of statistical, not identified, lives (Heinzerling 2000). The statistical nature of the lives protected by regulation of air toxics thus allows a reframing of the problem—to a problem of risk, not life—which itself allows—culturally, politically, morally—a pretty casual brush-off of the lives at stake.

A third kind of explanation for allowing pollution-related deaths combines both lives and costs in a cost-benefit framework and defends a choice not to protect lives by explaining that the deaths are not worth preventing in light of the costs of preventing them. As I have said, our environmental laws, for the most part, do not require, and often do not allow, a cost-benefit calculus in setting environmental standards. But executive orders on regulatory review going back to President Reagan have made cost-benefit analysis a dominant form of evaluating regulations even where it is not legally required or allowed (Heinzerling 2006b, 102). An important but little-known office within the White House, the Office of Information and Regulatory Affairs (OIRA), is responsible for reviewing significant regulations and blocking them if they are not up to snuff from the perspective of OIRA and the larger White House. As former OIRA administrator Cass Sunstein has acknowledged in his account of his time at OIRA, OIRA has not been shy about rejecting rules that do not pass its cost-benefit test (Sunstein 2013). (Anyone in doubt about the power of OIRA to stop rules should peruse OIRA's website (http://www.reginfo.gov), showing the many EPA rules that have been stuck at OIRA not only for months, but for years.)

Of course, where a statute forbids the consideration of costs, EPA may not explain a choice to save fewer lives on the grounds of costs. Likewise, where a statute requires a calculus different from cost-benefit analysis, EPA may not explain such a choice based on cost-benefit analysis. Yet if EPA wants its rules to come back from OIRA, it must be prepared to justify them to OIRA on the basis of cost-benefit analysis. This fact of the regulatory process has profound implications for the agency's approach to life-saving.

One result of the focus on cost-benefit analysis is that the statistical life, so respectfully treated in environmental laws as written, becomes easily expendable, easier to dismiss. The reason why cost-benefit analysis itself centers on the statistical life, rather than the identified life, is that the identified life often turns out to be priceless. If I asked you how much you would accept in money in exchange for my killing you, you would likely tell me to go away. You might even think I was a criminal. If I asked you how much you would pay me to avoid my killing you, you would likely tell me you would pay all you could afford (after threatening to have me arrested). Cost-benefit analysis of death-preventing measures breaks down in the face of the identified life; either no price will suffice, or the price will reflect—to an unusually dramatic extent—only ability to pay and not willingness to pay. Cost-benefit analysis has used the statistical life in order to render that life priceable (Heinzerling 2006a). Once the life has been priced—once it has been translated into dollars—it becomes fungible with any other priced item, and the anxiety we might experience in failing to come to the rescue of a fellow human being dissolves. In this way, the cost-benefit analysis required by the president and OIRA changes the thrust of environmental laws from fulsome protection to calculated forbearance.

Another result of the fixation on cost-benefit analysis is institutional. From the first moment EPA personnel conceive of a major rule, they begin to wonder: do the benefits of the rule justify the costs? In the case of life-saving rules, they wonder: will the rule prevent enough deaths to make the numbers work? In short, will OIRA let EPA issue this rule?

The power of OIRA over EPA rules turns the EPA analyst's mindset from the one envisioned in most environmental laws—to protect lives, even at great cost—to one in which there is sometimes quiet relief if costs can be trimmed even while lives are lost. Hundreds of lives become like so much pocket change when compared to billions of dollars in economic costs.

In these ways, the statistical life—despite its apparently high status in environmental law as written—turns out to be critical in softening the protections actually afforded by environmental law and, equally important, in skewing the mindset of the people trying to protect other people from environmental harms.

One lesson from this account is an old one: there is often a wide space between the aspirations of the law as written and the consequences of the law in practice. Another lesson is less familiar: it is exceedingly difficult to break out of the dichotomy between identified and statistical lives. Environmental laws have tried to do it; indeed, one plausible understanding of our environmental statutes is that they self-consciously reject the identifiable-victim focus of traditional tort law and acknowledge the moral claims of victims we cannot identify but who live and die, all the same. It is not an easy task, and the dichotomy persists.

One way to help decision-makers resist the temptation to dismiss the statistical life is to move from abstraction to concreteness in describing the consequences of pollution. One quite simple reform, already underway, is to report, in summary tables embedded in cost-benefit analyses, the actual number of lives saved through regulation and not just to report monetary values for them. Under its revised guidelines for economic analysis, issued in December 2010, EPA's Office of Policy instructs the agency's program offices to offer summary descriptions of regulatory benefits *"first in natural or physical units* (i.e., number) to provide a more complete picture of what the rule accomplishes" (EPA 2010, 11-3). Of course, this added bit of vivid detail comes in the midst of the analysis I have described as allowing the loss of statistical lives; but at least anyone reading the summary tables will know that human lives—and not just dollars—are at stake in the underlying decision. Another salutary reform would be to describe, in some detail, the actual physical consequences of the pollution under review. EPA should describe what bronchitis and asthma and cancer and the rest actually do to a body and a person and a life (Heinzerling 2011).

Another way of bringing home the tangible effects of pollution for real people, even if they are unidentified, would be to increase the granularity of information about the sources of health- and life-threatening pollution. People living in a neighborhood with a pollution source subject to an ongoing regulatory proceeding should be able to look up that source on a map and to learn about what concrete effects that source might have on their lives—and thus also to extrapolate to effects on others' lives, in other neighborhoods, faced with the same kinds of sources. EPA already offers some such information, by way of maps showing the locations of major sources of greenhouse gases (available at http://ghgdata.epa.gov/ghgp/main.do/); it should offer more.

In a quite different context, a federal trial court recently held that the residents of a neighborhood surrounding an oil refinery that had been operated in violation of federal environmental laws were entitled to be heard as crime victims under the Crime Victims' Rights Act (*United States v. CITGO Petroleum Corporation*, 2012 U.S. Dist. LEXIS 131,339 (S. Dist. Tex. 2012)). It is too early to tell exactly where this kind of proceeding will lead in terms of rendering the consequences of pollution in vivid enough detail to break out of the dichotomy between identified and statistical lives. But it—along with the other reforms I have mentioned—is a start.

One of the great triumphs of US environmental law is its aspiration to prevent future harms. In this achievement there also lies a challenge. The future-oriented, preventative thrust of environmental law means that its preoccupation is the statistical, not identified, life. The statistical life is easy to bury: in economic costs, in calculations of risk, in cost-benefit comparisons. I have suggested that one way out of this dilemma is to bring statistical lives into focus as vividly as possible through detailed descriptions of the harms wrought by pollution.

Acknowledgment

This chapter draws in part on the author's experiences while at the Environmental Protection Agency.

References

Adler, Matthew D. 2005. "Against 'Individual Risk': A Sympathetic Critique of Risk Assessment." *University of Pennsylvania Law Review* 153: 1121–250.
Administration of Barack Obama. 2011. "Statement on the Ozone National Ambient Air Quality Standards." September 2. Daily Comp. Pres. Docs. 201100607. Available from http://www.whitehouse.gov/the-press-office/2011/09/02/statement-president-ozone-national-ambient-air-quality-standards/.
Broder, John M. 2011. "Re-election Strategy Is Tied to a Shift on Smog." *New York Times*. November 17, Page A1.

Environmental Protection Agency (EPA). 2009. "Risk and Technology Review (RTR) Risk Assessment Methodologies: For Review by the EPA's Science Advisory Board." June. Available from http://www.epa.gov/ttn/atw/rrisk/rtrpg.html/.
———. 2010. "Guidelines for Preparing Economic Analysis." December.
———. 2011. "Regulatory Impact Analysis, Final National Ambient Air Quality Standards for Ozone." July. Available from http://www.epa.gov/glo/pdfs/201107_OMBdraft-OzoneRIA.pdf.
Heinzerling, Lisa. 2000. "The Rights of Statistical People." *Harvard Environmental Law Review* 24: 189–207.
———. 2006a. "Knowing Killing and Environmental Law." *New York University Environmental Law Journal* 14: 521–34.
———. 2006b. "Statutory Interpretation in the Era of OIRA." *Fordham Urban Law Journal* 33: 1097–117.
———. 2011. "Missing a Teachable Moment: The Obama Administration and the Importance of Regulation." American Constitution Society Issue Brief.
Lewis, Michael. 2012. "Obama's Way." *Vanity Fair*, October.
Sunstein, Cass R. 2013. *Simpler: The Future of Government*. New York: Simon & Schuster.

13 }

Treatment versus Prevention in the Fight against HIV/AIDS and the Problem of Identified versus Statistical Lives

Johann Frick

1. Introduction

For years, discussions about the best way to combat the HIV/AIDS pandemic have pitted proponents of scaling up antiretroviral treatment for people already suffering from AIDS against other writers, who advocate for a focus on more cost-effective prevention measures. In an important recent article, Dan Brock and Daniel Wikler (2009) frame the underlying moral issue as a debate about whether, given long-term budget constraints, there are any moral grounds to privilege the saving of identified lives through antiretroviral treatment, even if concentrating on preventive methods could save more (statistical) lives overall.

In this chapter, I critically examine Brock and Wikler's contention that since all human lives have equal worth, there can be no sound moral basis for giving any priority to the saving of identified over statistical lives, all else equal. In so doing, I develop a novel account of how the choice between "treatment" and "prevention" in population-level health policy intersects the problem of identified versus statistical lives. The chapter concludes with a postscript on "treatment-as-prevention," a new avenue of AIDS research that stresses the preventive benefits of early antiretroviral treatment. I argue that, while scientifically promising, treatment-as-prevention does not transcend the ethical dichotomy between treatment and prevention explored in this chapter.

2. Brock and Wikler's Argument

Human beings have a well-documented psychological propensity to attach greater importance to rescuing identified individuals from imminent peril than to preventing the loss of statistical lives.[1] By "statistical lives," I mean lives that will predictably be lost to known risk factors in the future unless we intervene, but whose identities it is impossible for us to know, at least at present[2] (and sometimes even in hindsight).[3]

However, is this propensity anything more than an empirical fact about how we tend to behave? Is there any reason to believe that it also corresponds, at least under certain conditions, to what we have moral reason to do? In recent years, many economists, philosophers, and lawyers have greeted this idea with skepticism.[4]

Brock and Wikler (2009) are a prominent example of this trend. Noting that despite recent increases in funding for antiretroviral treatment the goal of achieving universal access to treatment seems unlikely to be achieved in the foreseeable future, Brock and Wikler advocate for scaling back expensive antiretroviral treatment for people suffering from HIV/AIDS in favor of preventive interventions (educational campaigns, male medical circumcision, condom distribution, etc.), which promise to save more lives overall (see, e.g., Marseille, Hoffman, and Kahn 2002). Since we cannot know in advance, nor

---

[1] The labels "identified" and "statistical" lives are due to Schelling (1968). For empirical studies of the "identified victims effect," see Moore (1996) and Jenni and Loewenstein (1997).

[2] Note that this way of drawing the distinction between identified and statistical lives makes the distinction nonexhaustive. Alongside identified lives, whose identities we do know at present, and statistical lives, whose identities we cannot know at present but only once they have been lost (and sometimes not even then: see the following note), there are also what one might call "identifiable lives." These are lives whose identities we do not currently know, but which we could come to know before they are lost, using presently available evidence and/or scientific know-how. Suppose 50 miners are trapped underground. We may not currently know their names, but we could easily find out (e.g., by checking to see which miners are missing). These lives are identifiable. Similarly, suppose a virus threatens all and only those members of the population with blood type AB+. If we do not know who has that blood type, the lives threatened by the virus are not identified lives. But by conducting a simple blood test, we could identify them. Although, for simplicity of exposition, I shall largely focus on the conventional distinction between identified and statistical lives in this chapter, much of what I say about the special moral reasons for saving identified lives (over statistical lives) would apply to identifiable lives as well. I briefly return to this issue in note 10 below.

[3] That we often cannot know, even in hindsight, the identities of those statistical lives who were affected by our action is true both for cases where these lives were saved, as well as for cases where these lives were lost. Take the latter case first: Suppose a nuclear power plant very slightly raises the risk that each person living in its vicinity has of dying from cancer. At the aggregate level, the presence of the nuclear power plant foreseeably results in a somewhat higher level of cancer deaths in the surrounding population than would otherwise have been the case. At the same time, it may be impossible to state which individual cancer deaths are causally attributable to the power plant (in the sense that they would not have occurred in the absence of the power plant), and which would have occurred anyway. Similarly, suppose that treating a community's drinking water reduces the number of statistical lives lost to waterborne diseases. Must it be the case that there is even a fact of the matter about who would have lost her life, had the drinking water been left untreated, and hence about whose life we saved? Even if there was such a fact of the matter, there is no reason to think that we could know it.

[4] For two seminal discussions, see Schelling (1968) and Fried (1969). For a rare recent argument in defense of giving priority to the saving of identified lives, see Norman Daniels (2012).

probably even in hindsight, whose life will be saved by such prevention measures, the loss of life averted in this way is statistical.

Brock and Wikler write:

> When resources do not permit all to be saved, it is better to save more lives than fewer, provided that the beneficiaries are chosen fairly—all other things held equal. If prevention would save more lives, it is the better choice from a moral point of view—again, if all other things held equal. (Brock and Wikler 2009, 1668)

But are all other things equal? The most serious moral objection that Brock and Wikler consider is that shifting money away from treating existing AIDS sufferers into prevention is morally impermissible because it violates the "Rule of Rescue." According to this ethical principle, "the fact that we can save identified people whose lives are imminently threatened by AIDS creates an obligation to do so that must be honored even if doing so reduces the number of lives saved overall" (Brock and Wikler 2009, 1670).

Brock and Wikler reject the Rule of Rescue, at least as it applies to the battle against HIV/AIDS. Although they are willing to allow that principles of nonabandonment may have a place in the role morality of medical doctors, who have face-to-face interactions and relationships of trust with individual patients, they insist that the distinction between identified and statistical lives has no moral relevance for population-level bioethics—the level at which strategic decisions in the global struggle against HIV/AIDS are taken: "Put most simply, statistical lives are just as real as identified lives saved; all have the same equal worth" (Brock and Wikler 2009, 1671).

Even outside the sphere of bioethics, Brock and Wikler think our much greater preparedness to expend resources to save, rather than to prevent, lives from being lost frequently leads to irrational results. For instance, in most societies "no resources will be spared to try to rescue trapped miners ... even if [less costly] safety measures that would have prevented the cave-in were deemed too expensive the previous year" (Brock and Wikler 2009, 1670).

There is no doubt that the dispositions that Brock and Wikler allude to often do lead to irrational behavior. In their mining example, if our propensity to give greater salience to the prevention of identified losses causes us to wait until a cave-in has occurred and then rescue those trapped in the mine, rather than prevent the disaster by expending fewer resources earlier on, this is a costly form of moral myopia. It is akin to the hyperbolic discounting studied by decision theorists, which fuels procrastination and other forms of irrational behavior. I also do not wish to dispute Brock and Wikler's claim that statistical and identified lives have equal worth—a point that seems to me obviously correct.

My reservation about Brock and Wikler's argument stems from the fact that I am not convinced that they have met their self-imposed argumentative burden, namely to show that shifting resources from the treatment to prevention will not be "unfair" to those already suffering from HIV/AIDS.

My argument in the following will rest on two principal ideas: (1) skepticism about interpersonal aggregation and (2) the proposition that, all else equal, individuals have a stronger claim to be protected from some harm, the greater their likelihood of suffering that harm. I shall introduce these two ideas in turn, before making a first pass at presenting my argument.

3. Competing Claims and the Distinction between Identified and Statistical Lives

There are some ethical theories according to which the distinction between identified and statistical lives is devoid of moral significance. The most prominent such view is act-consequentialism, which holds that the rightness of an action is determined solely by the goodness of the state of affairs that it produces (or can be expected to produce). According to the act-consequentialist, an act is right just if its consequences are at least as good as those of any other available alternative act. Since, as Brock and Wikler emphasize, a statistical life is "just as real" as that of an identified person, preventing it from being lost contributes just as much to the goodness of an action's consequences as the saving of an identified life.[5] If, therefore, we could avert more loss of life by focusing on prevention than by rescuing the lives of identified persons through treatment, this is the course of action that act-consequentialism would require of us.

Act-consequentialism, however, is far from being an uncontroversial moral theory. Many of the strongest objections to act-consequentialism focus on its embrace of *interpersonal aggregation*: According to the act-consequentialist, in evaluating an action we should morally sum the benefits and losses it imposes on different persons to obtain an aggregate quantity; this characterizes the overall goodness of the action's consequences. The rightness or wrongness of the action is a function, not of how it treats each individual, but of the net balance of benefits over losses.

Aggregative reasoning of this kind frequently yields counterintuitive implications, especially where the benefits or harms to different people are very different in size. Consider:

> *Life versus Headaches*: We could either save Fred's life or prevent one million people from suffering a headache.

---

[5] In the following I assume, for the sake of simplicity, that the identical and statistical lives in question are alike in all morally relevant respects. In particular, I assume that by saving a statistical life, we allow the person to live on for the same number of years, at an equivalent quality of life, as we would by saving the life of an identified person. Hence, the number of QALYs preserved by saving either life is the same.

Many of us have the intuition that it would be wrong not to save Fred's life regardless of how many people's headaches we could prevent instead. The harm of a headache is trivial compared to that of losing one's life. No matter how large the sum of these harms, we think, it would be wrong to let Fred lose his life in order to prevent them.[6] Defenders of interpersonal aggregation, by contrast, are committed to the position that there must be some point (if not at one million people, then at some higher number) at which preventing the headaches of the many morally outweighs saving Fred from death.

A common nonconsequentialist diagnosis for the inadequacy of aggregative views is that they fail to respect what, following John Rawls, is often referred to as "the separateness of persons" (Rawls 1999, 167). Collections of people are not super-individuals. Unlike a single individual, who may rationally choose to make some sacrifice now in exchange for receiving a stream of benefits later on, a group of people lacks the requisite unity such that imposing a significant harm on one person could be straightforwardly offset by giving sufficient benefits to others. The relations between different persons are not like those between different temporal parts of a life.

As a better way of respecting the separateness of persons, leading nonconsequentialists have argued for a different way of evaluating the rightness of our actions. According to the so-called "competing claims" model of moral rightness (sometimes also referred to as the "complaint" model), morality requires us to determine that action or policy which satisfies the strongest individual claim or (what amounts to the same thing) minimizes the strongest complaint had by any individual (where complaints are what individuals have just in case their individual claims are not satisfied) (see, e.g., Scanlon 1998, ch. 5; see also Temkin 2012, ch. 3; and Nagel 1991). The competing claims model yields the intuitively correct verdict about the *Life versus Headaches* case. Since Fred has a much stronger claim to be saved from death than any individual has to be spared a headache, we ought to save Fred.

At first blush, however, it may seem that skepticism about interpersonal aggregation ought to have little bearing on the problem of identified versus statistical lives. After all, unlike in the *Life versus Headaches* example, cases where we must decide between saving some number of identified lives or a greater number of statistical lives are ones where what is at stake for the persons on either side of the trade-off is a harm of equivalent seriousness: losing their life. But surely, even if we are skeptical about interpersonal aggregation in general, we ought to accept that, when faced with a choice between saving a smaller or a greater number of lives, we ought to save the greater number.

---

[6] Philosophers who have defended this view include Scanlon (1998, 235); Kamm (2009, 155); and Temkin (2012, 36).

Most nonconsequentialists do indeed accept this, at least when what is at stake for the people in either group is certain death.[7] But it is precisely in this respect that the problem of identified versus statistical lives differs from the standard "numbers" problem, in a way that I shall argue is morally significant.

Saving an identified person from death means saving someone who, but for our intervention (or that of someone else), was certain (or at least very likely) to die. By contrast, the way in which we prevent the loss of statistical lives is, typically, by reducing or eliminating the risk of death faced by each member of some larger group. Suppose, for instance, that one million people each face a 1 in 1,000 risk of death, and that these risks are probabilistically independent. Although the risk of death to each person is small, due to the law of large numbers it is a statistical certainty that some people will lose their lives; moreover, we can predict with a high degree of confidence that the number of deaths will equal roughly 1,000. By decreasing the risk of death for each person by 10%, to 9 in 10,000, we can expect to save 100 statistical lives. The important takeaway from this example is that saving a statistical life often comes about by slightly reducing a risk of death to many people that was already quite small to begin with.

This distinction, between preventing loss of life by saving people from almost certain death versus preventing loss of life by slightly reducing the risk of death for many people, whose antecedent chance of death was already significantly smaller, is mirrored in the choice between treatment and prevention: without access to antiretroviral drugs, persons who currently suffer from AIDS are almost certain to die within a short period of time; on the other hand, prevention measures merely serve to further reduce a given uninfected person's much lower risk of contracting and dying from AIDS in the future.

This difference, I claim, is morally significant. Like some other philosophers (for instance, Norman Daniels, in this volume), I believe that individuals have a stronger claim to be protected from a harm that they would otherwise suffer with certainty than from a mere risk of suffering a harm of equivalent size. For instance, given a choice between saving A from certain death or protecting B from a 20% risk of death, A has a much stronger claim to be protected than B. (Call this the *One versus One* case.) The reason for this is that a person has a much stronger prudential interest in avoiding certain death than a mere 20% chance of death.[8] This is not to say, of course, that if

---

[7] Philosophers like John Taurek (1977), who deny that there is any obligation to save the greater number, are very much in the minority, even in the nonconsequentialist camp. T. M. Scanlon, for instance, argues that when harms of equivalent seriousness are at stake, numbers act to "break the tie." See Scanlon (1998, 232), following the argument in Kamm (1993, 116–17).

[8] Note, incidentally, that this is true whether the 20% risk in question stems from a deterministic or an indeterministic causal process. If the causal process is indeterministic, B has a 20% objective chance of dying. If the causal process is deterministic, B's 20% risk of death is *epistemic*, i.e., due not to indeterminacy at the level of physical reality itself, but to our incomplete knowledge of the state of the

B is unlucky and her 20% risk of death materializes, she will not lose just as much as A would, if we left him to his certain death. The claim is merely that, since B is less likely to suffer this bad fate than A, her claim to our assistance is comparatively weaker.

4. The Pro Identified Lives Argument and Its Discontents

We are now in a position to see how the two moral ideas I have just sketched—skepticism about interpersonal aggregation and the thought that people have a weaker claim to be saved from mere risks as opposed to certain harms—together lend support to the idea that we may have moral reason to privilege the saving of identified over statistical lives.

Consider the following *Pro Identified Lives Argument*.

I have just argued that

(1) In the *One versus One* case, given a choice between saving A from certain death or protecting B from a 20% risk of death, A has a much stronger claim to be saved than B. Correspondingly, A would have a much stronger complaint if we saved B than B would have if we saved A.

Consider now the following choice:

One versus Five: We have to choose between saving A from certain death and protecting each of C, D, E, F, and G from a 20% risk of death. (Assume that the risks to each of the five are probabilistically independent. We expect that not eliminating the risk to C, D, E, F, and G will result in the death of one of them—though there may also be zero deaths, or more than one. However, we have no way of knowing who will die if we do not protect C, D, E, F, and G from their 20% risk of death. The expected losses are thus statistical.)

It seems true that

(2) In the *One versus Five* case, C, D, E, F, or G—considered as individuals—would be treated no differently, if we decided to save A, than was B in the *One versus One* case. That is, they would each remain

---

world and the laws of nature. Given the available evidence, there is a 20% epistemic chance that the causal process is objectively certain to kill B and an 80% epistemic chance that it is objectively certain not to kill her. However, in both the deterministic and the indeterministic case, B's rational degree of credence that she will avoid death is the same, namely 0.8. From the perspective of prudential self-interest, this is all that matters, I believe. That is, as far as the justifiability of our action to B is concerned, it makes no difference whether the 20% risk of death that B is exposed to is objective or epistemic. For a more detailed discussion of this question, see my manuscript "Contractualism and Social Risk: How to Count the Numbers without Aggregating" (available on request).

exposed to a 20% risk of death when they could instead have had their risk of death reduced to zero.

Hence, it seems plausible to assert that

(3) In the *One versus Five* case, none of C, D, E, F, or G has a stronger individual claim to be protected from their 20% risk of death than B has in the *One versus One* case.

Furthermore, as we saw above, many nonconsequentialists accept the following principle:

(4) In deciding which course of action to pursue, we must not combine or aggregate the claims of different individuals. Rather, according to the competing claims model, we should select that action which satisfies the strongest individual claim.

But from (1), (3), and (4) it follows that

(5) In the *One versus Five* case, we ought to save A from certain death, rather than protect C, D, E, F, and G from a 20% risk of death, since this is what satisfies the strongest individual claim. A would have a stronger complaint if we decided to protect C, D, E, F, and G from their 20% risk of death than any of these individuals would have if we saved A from certain death.

If the Pro Identified Lives Argument is sound, it would provide a justification for privileging the saving of identified over that of statistical lives in many cases. On this account, the distinction between identified and statistical lives is often morally relevant, when and because it coincides with that between saving those who are certain (or very likely) to die unless we intervene, and those who face a smaller individual risk of death.

There is a sense, however, in which the Pro Identified Lives Argument succeeds too well. Notice that its conclusion is not at all sensitive to the total number of statistical deaths that we allow to happen by saving A from certain death. Suppose that instead of five there had been 50 people whom we could have protected from having each to face a 20% risk of death. (Call this the *One versus 50* case.) Here, choosing to save A will result in approximately 10 statistical deaths. The Pro Identified Lives Argument, however, is impervious to this fact: As long as A's claim to be saved from certain death is stronger than that of any of the 50 individuals to be spared their 20% chance of death, the logic of the argument compels us to save A.

Most people will find this conclusion hard to stomach. It seems acceptable, even conforms to most people's intuition, to give somewhat greater weight to the saving of identified over that of statistical lives (so that we might prefer to save A from certain death rather than protect, say, eight individuals from each facing a 20% risk of death) (the *One versus Eight* case). However, a view that would, in principle, allow us to let any number of statistical lives be lost in order to save one identified individual from certain death seems deeply implausible.

5. The Ex Ante versus the Ex Post View

Let us, then, consider ways in which this unpalatable conclusion might be avoided.

One option I have already canvassed above: If we jettisoned nonconsequentialist strictures on aggregation, thus rejecting premise (4) of the Pro Identified Lives Argument, this would allow us to say the following: while C, D, E, F, and G may each have a lesser individual claim to be spared their 20% risk of death, pooling these claims can yield a combined claim that is equivalent in strength to A's claim to be saved from certain death. Moreover, in the *One versus 50* case, the combined claim of the 50 would far exceed that of A. While this proposal differs from standard consequentialism by making the right a function of the combined claims of individuals rather than of aggregate goodness, its prescriptions would be extensionally equivalent to those of act-consequentialism. As such, it would place no special weight on the saving of identified lives.

Like act-consequentialism, however, this view must contend with problem cases like *Life versus Headaches* above. If we concede that the weaker individual claims of many may be morally summed and can together overcome the weighty claim of one individual in the *One versus 50* case, do we have the resources to block the same kind of move in *Life versus Headaches*, where it would have very unattractive implications? It is not clear to me that we do.

There may, however, be a different way of avoiding the conclusion of the Pro Identified Lives Argument, without leaving the framework of the competing claims model. Instead of jettisoning premise (4) above, we might challenge premise (3) instead. Premise (3) implicitly relies on a view—call it the *ex ante view*—according to which the strength of a person's claim to be protected from a risk of harm (and the seriousness of her complaint if she is not), is a function of the size of the harm discounted by her own ex ante likelihood of suffering the harm.

Someone might object to this ex ante view as follows: "In a case like *One versus Five*, it seems morally irrelevant that we cannot know in advance who of C, D, E, F, or G will end up dying if we decide to save A instead. What matters, rather, is that we know that one of them will die if we save A. That is, one of the five will end up just as badly off if we do not protect the five as will A if we do not save him. There is thus nothing to choose between either course of action in the *One versus Five* case. We might as well flip a coin. Moreover, in the *One versus 50* case, where saving A will foreseeably result in 10 statistical deaths, we morally ought to protect the 10 from their 20% risk of death rather than save A, since when individual claims of equal weight are at stake, even the competing claims model tells us to save the greater number."

A proponent of this objection to the Pro Identified Lives Argument endorses what I call the *ex post view*. According to this view, the strength of a person's claim to be protected from a risk of harm (and the seriousness of her complaint if she is not), depends not on how likely she herself was to suffer a harm, but only on how likely it was that *someone* would. As Sophia Reibetanz Moreau, a defender of the ex post view writes:

> As long as we know that acceptance of a principle will affect *someone* in a certain way, we should assign that person a complaint that is based upon the full magnitude of the harm or benefit, even if we cannot identify the person in advance. It is only if we do not know whether acceptance of a principle will affect anyone in a certain way that we should allocate each individual a complaint based upon his expected harms and benefits under that principle.[9]

The ex post view promises to avoid the excessive disregard for the protection of statistical lives that the ex ante view entails. Indeed, as long as it is certain that a given course of action will lead to statistical lives being lost, the ex post view accords these statistical victims an individual complaint just as weighty as that of identified victims.

6. Why the Ex Post View Must Be Rejected

Unfortunately, the ex post view faces its own set of problems that, I will argue, are even more serious as those confronting the ex ante view.

For one thing, notice that there is an odd tension in the ex post view: a proponent of the ex post view concedes that in the *One versus One* case, B's complaint about being left exposed to a 20% risk of death is much weaker than the complaint that A would have if we did not save him from certain death. By contrast, in a case like *One versus Five*, the ex post view holds that, whoever of the five turns out to be harmed, that person would have a complaint almost as strong as A's, despite the fact that her own risk of harm was no greater than that of B in the *One versus One* case. Somehow, the fact that, if we save A, it is very likely that someone from the group of five will be harmed, is supposed to enhance the complaint of whoever turns out to be harmed.

But why should this be the case, exactly? Suppose C is the unlucky one. Why should C's complaint be any greater than B's in the *One versus Five* case, just because, had C not been harmed, some other person from the group of five would have been harmed instead? This looks suspiciously like a tacit appeal to a new form of interpersonal aggregation: the combination of complaints by different individuals at different possible worlds, depending on who happens

---

[9] Reibetanz Moreau (1998, 304). Michael Otsuka (in this volume) also defends a view of this type.

to be unlucky at that possible world. But if nonconsequentialists reject the combination of claims by different people at the same possible world, then ought they not, a fortiori, to bar different individuals from aggregating their complaints across different possible worlds?

Second, there are many cases in which the ex post view would dramatically contradict our ordinary moral convictions. Consider:

> *Mass Vaccination*: We vaccinate 100 million children against some serious, but nonfatal childhood disease, which each of these children is otherwise certain to contract. The vast majority of children will benefit from the protection the vaccination offers. However, for every child there is also a very remote possibility of fatal side effects from the vaccination itself. Specifically, we foresee that there will be roughly 100 statistical deaths as a result of the vaccination drive.

Although this example is highly stylized, cases with a structure that is similar in morally relevant respects are very common in everyday life. That is, in pursuit of moderate benefits for many people, we routinely engage in risky actions or policies that will foreseeably result in severe harms befalling a few statistical victims. (Think of higher speed limits on motorways, large-scale construction projects, vaccination drives, etc.). Nonetheless, such instances of "social risk" are commonly deemed morally innocuous. Indeed, without the license to engage in actions or policies of this type, social life would grind to a halt.

In the above case, it is not hard to see why a policy of vaccinating every child is intuitively permissible. Receiving the vaccination can be justified to each child as being in her own interest: avoiding the burden of a serious childhood illness, most would agree, is worth a tiny, one in a million risk of death. It is true that there will foreseeably be some statistical loss of life. But this comes about through a process that was exceedingly unlikely to harm any given child. The ex ante view, by discounting the complaints of statistical victims by their unlikelihood, captures this intuition.

By contrast, if the ex post view were correct, instances of social risk-imposition like *Mass Vaccination* would be morally indefensible. Given that we know in advance that there is sure to be some statistical loss of life if we vaccinate, the ex post view implies that we must not discount the harm-based complaints of the statistical victims. But, of course, a person's undiscounted complaint against premature death is much greater than any individual's complaint against suffering a nonfatal childhood disease. Hence, the only permissible course of action, according to a competing claims model informed by the ex post view, is not to vaccinate.

This is not only the intuitively wrong answer. Even more damagingly, the ex post view also lacks the resources to recognize the moral difference between cases like *Mass Vaccination* and the following case:

> *Water Supply*: Everything is as in *Mass Vaccination* above, except that this time we know in advance which children will die as a result of being

vaccinated and which will benefit. However, the only way of vaccinating the children who will benefit is by vaccinating those who will be harmed as well. For instance, assume (somewhat fancifully) that the only way of distributing the vaccine to any child is by putting it in the general water supply that all children must drink from.

Vaccinating all 100 million children in *Water Supply* would amount to sacrificing the lives of a small number of identified children in order to spare the other children the burden of a nonfatal childhood disease. This, clearly, is much more morally problematic. The problem for the ex post view is that it must regard *Mass Vaccination* and *Water Supply* as being morally on a par. That is, it is committed to conflating the moral significance of the following two propositions:

(1) It is certain that some children will die if we vaccinate, which is true in both *Vaccination* and *Water Supply*; and
(2) There are some children who are certain to die if we vaccinate, which is true only in the latter case.

According to the ex post view, as long as we know that (1) is true, it is morally irrelevant whether (2) is also true or not. The fact that in *Water Supply* we know from the start that our policy will kill a specific group of children, whereas in *Mass Vaccination* it will merely impose on each child a minuscule risk of death, is deemed to be morally irrelevant. This is very implausible.[10]

Act-consequentialism, incidentally, faces the same problem in the reverse direction: By assumption, the overall outcome of vaccinating, that is, the number

---

[10] Consider, briefly, what changes if the lives that will be lost in *Water Supply* are not identified, but merely identifiable, in the sense of note 2 above. Suppose that we know that the vaccine will benefit all children, except those that carry a certain, highly rare gene, which we are able to easily and reliably detect. All children with this gene will be killed by the vaccine. However, although we know that roughly 100 out of the 100 million affected children carry the gene, we do not currently know their identities. Does this matter morally? Would vaccinating be morally less problematic in this revised version of *Water Supply* (call it *Water Supply**) than in the original case with identified victims? I do not think it would be. The crucial moral difference between *Mass Vaccination* and the original *Water Supply* case is that only in the former case can we say to each child that, to the very best of our knowledge, receiving the vaccine is highly likely to benefit her, and has only a tiny chance of harming her. We would give her the vaccine even in a single-person case, where furthering her interests was our sole concern. By contrast, in both *Water Supply* and *Water Supply** we know that there are some children who are certain to die if they receive the vaccine. The only difference between *Water Supply* and *Water Supply** is that in the original case we already know these "doomed" children's identities, whereas in the revised case we could easily come to know them by finding out which children carry the rare gene. But surely, if vaccinating would be unjustifiable in *Water Supply*, because we already know the identities of the doomed children, ignorance of the doomed children's identities would be a very poor excuse for vaccinating in *Water Supply**. For this lack of information about the doomed children's identities is one that we are entirely free to remove. Saying to each child in *Water Supply** that "to the very best of our knowledge" she will benefit from receiving the vaccine would thus be disingenuous, in a way that it would not be in *Mass Vaccination*, where we have no way of knowing in advance who will benefit and who will be harmed by the vaccine.

of children benefited and harmed, will be the same in *Mass Vaccination* and *Water Supply*. Hence, if the consequentialist deems vaccination to be morally permissible in *Mass Vaccination*—because the aggregate benefit of protecting close to 100 million children from a serious childhood disease outweighs the aggregate harm to the unlucky 100 who die from side effects—the same must be true in *Water Supply* as well. But this, again, is a deeply unattractive conclusion.[11]

Might the force of my argument in support of the ex ante view be evaded by invoking a moral distinction between harming and not aiding a person? According to some nonconsequentialist moral philosophers, our reasons against imposing some loss on a person are often more stringent than our reasons against allowing a person to suffer a loss of equivalent size by not aiding her.[12] Furthermore, it is true that if we choose to vaccinate in *Water Supply*, we will harm some children (in the sense of actively imposing losses on them), whereas failing to vaccinate and allowing all children to contract the childhood disease would merely constitute a failure to aid. Might this, rather than the ex ante view, provide the correct explanation of why it seems morally problematic to vaccinate in *Water Supply*, but not in *Mass Vaccination*?[13]

This explanation will not work. Notice that in terms of the harming/not aiding distinction, the two options in *Mass Vaccination* are exactly parallel to those in *Water Supply*: if we proceed with the vaccination, we will foreseeably harm 100 statistical individuals, causing them to lose their lives. By contrast, if we do nothing, we allow 100 million children to suffer a serious childhood disease, which constitutes a failure to aid. Thus, even if there is a morally relevant distinction between harming and not aiding, this distinction by itself cannot explain our divergent intuitions about *Mass Vaccination* and *Water Supply*—namely that it would be comparatively morally innocuous to vaccinate in the former case, whereas doing so in the latter would be deeply morally problematic. In order to do so, we need something like the ex ante view.

7. Toward a Pluralist Account of Moral Rightness

Here is where we stand: As we just saw, an ethical theory that treats the loss of statistical lives as morally equivalent to the loss of identified lives robs itself of the ability to distinguish between intuitively permissible instances of social risk, like *Mass Vaccination*, and morally impermissible trade-offs, like *Water Supply*. This is a strike against both the ex post view and act-consequentialism.

---

[11] For a more detailed argument against the ex post view, see my "Contractualism and Social Risk: How to Count the Numbers without Aggregating" (n.d.). See also Frick (2013).

[12] For a helpful discussion, see Kamm (2007, ch. 1).

[13] I thank an anonymous referee for raising this objection.

The ex ante view, by contrast, avoids this problem, but faces its own difficulties in cases like *One versus 50* in section 4 above. Is there a way out of this impasse?

I believe that there is, once we drop the assumption that our only choice is act-consequentialism or a pure competing claims model (be it one that incorporates the ex ante or the ex post view). Instead, I propose that we ought to adopt a *pluralist* account of moral rightness.

I believe that the ex ante version of the competing claims model must form part of this pluralist view if we are to explain the clear intuitive difference between cases like *Mass Vaccination* and *Water Supply*. We thus ought to accept, contra the ex post view, that even in cases where it is foreseeable that some people will end up being harmed, the strength of an individual's claims against being exposed to harm must be discounted by her own ex ante probability of suffering harm.

On the other hand, cases like *One versus 50* force us to acknowledge that a pure competing claims model informed by the ex ante view does not render the correct all-things-considered verdict in all situations either.

To escape this dilemma, we ought to embrace a pluralist position, according to which satisfying the strongest individual claim had by any person is one, but not the only relevant consideration in evaluating whether an action is right all things considered. Rather than providing an account of moral rightness all things considered, the competing claims model, on this view, captures an important class of pro tanto reasons, compliance with which contributes to making actions right or wrong all things considered. For lack of a better term, we might say that the moral reasons captured by the competing claims model are ones of *fairness*. It is unfair to let Fred lose his life so that other people may be spared the much smaller harm of a headache; and likewise it is unfair to leave A exposed to certain death, so that others may avoid a much smaller risk of death. However, in determining whether a course of action is morally right all things considered, the aims given to us by the competing claims model must sometimes be traded off against other considerations—importantly among them, pro tanto reasons to be concerned with the consequences in terms of people's well-being that our action produces. In some cases, such as *Mass Vaccination*, these two sets of pro tanto reasons point in the same direction; in others, like *One versus 50*, they pull in opposite directions.[14]

Giving fairness its due means that in a case like *One versus Five*, where the two possible actions do not differ in terms of their expected consequences (we expect one person to die whichever option we choose), reasons of fairness determine that we ought to save A's identified life, since this will satisfy the strongest individual claim. Likewise, when two options do not differ by

---

[14] For a somewhat similar account, according to which fairness consists in satisfying people's claims in proportion to their strength, but must sometimes be traded off against other considerations, see Broome (1990, 1994).

much in terms of their expected consequences, as in the *One versus Eight* case, reasons of fairness may outweigh a concern with people's well-being. By contrast, when the difference in the expected consequences is as large as in *One versus 50*, it is plausible that any concern with fairness is swamped by our well-being-given reasons for averting an outcome in which many more lives are lost.[15]

Somewhere in between these extremes, there is a tipping point at which reasons of fairness begin to be outweighed by well-being-given reasons. I cannot tell you where exactly this tipping point is located, nor can I provide you with a general algorithm by which to determine the relative weight to be placed on fairness and well-being in other cases. But nor do I think it is my role to do so. The aim and ambition of moral philosophy is to inform our moral judgment, by making us alive to the relevant ethical considerations, not to abolish the need for judgment.

8. The Importance of Temporal Structure

It is time to return to the problem of treatment versus prevention in the fight against HIV/AIDS. If my argument in the previous sections is sound, Brock and Wikler are wrong to claim that, given the equal worth of all human lives, there could be no morally relevant difference between saving identified lives through treatment and averting the loss of statistical lives through prevention.

If we do not treat people already suffering from HIV/AIDS, they will soon die with near certainty. By contrast, failing to undertake all the preventive efforts at our disposal means that uninfected persons will be at a somewhat

---

[15] Of course, this sketched solution leaves many details to be filled in. For instance, what exactly determines the strength of our well-being-given reasons for choosing one option over another? The answer depends, in part, on the appropriate aggregative procedure for combining the well-being-given reasons that we have for helping different individuals. In a situation like *Life versus Headaches*, must it be the case, as act-consequentialists assume, that the very weak well-being-given reasons that we have for preventing each of the million individuals from suffering a headache together give us a stronger reason of well-being than our weighty well-being-given reason for saving Fred's life? It is not clear to me that they do. Following Frances Kamm's suggestion in *Intricate Ethics*, I believe that, in a context where we have weighty well-being-given reasons to prevent someone from suffering a serious harm, the much weaker well-being-given reasons to prevent other individuals from suffering a very minor harm are not "relevant," and cannot together outweigh the well-being-given reasons to prevent the serious harm (see Kamm 2007, 34–35 and 384–85). If this were the case, then saving Fred's life would be the right thing to do, not just because it satisfies the reasons of fairness captured by the competing claims model, but also because it is what we have most well-being-given reasons to do. Unfortunately, I do not have the space to pursue these questions further here. In the following, I merely rely on the very plausible assumption that, when what is at stake for individuals on both sides of the trade-off are harms or losses of the same (or closely similar) magnitude, as is the case when deciding whether to prevent the loss of identified or statistical lives, we have most well-being-given reason to do what will save the largest number of lives.

higher risk of contracting, and dying from, AIDS in the future. But even in countries with very high prevalence of AIDS, this risk will be much lower than 100%—indeed, in all but the very worst-affected countries, it falls below the 20% figure that I have been using in most of my examples. Therefore, if people have a stronger claim to be protected from certain death than to have their risk of death further reduced, this gives us at least a pro tanto reason of fairness for giving some preference to saving identified lives through treatment rather than statistical lives through prevention.

Of course, how heavily this consideration ought to weigh in our-all-things-considered judgment will depend on how large a discrepancy there is between the numbers of lives we save by focusing on prevention as opposed to treatment. If the discrepancy is very large, it may be that any concern with fairness or people's individual claims is swamped by our well-being-given reasons for saving many more lives.

There is one more complexity to be considered. Note that the bioethicist's dichotomy between "treatment" and "prevention" need only partially overlap with that between saving "identified" versus "statistical" lives. Focusing on "treatment," in particular, might mean two quite different things:

(1) using the resources at our disposal to treat people currently suffering from AIDS;
(2) using the resources at our disposal to invest in the means to treat people suffering from AIDS at some future time.

To see why this ambiguity in the term "treatment" is morally significant, consider the following case:

> *Policymaker's Trilemma*: Suppose a health policymaker must decide between the following three ways of spending the funds available to his district for fighting AIDS:
>
> - *Present Treatment*: Spend all available funds to save the lives of 500 identified persons currently suffering from AIDS in his district.
> - *Future Treatment*: Spend all available funds to enable better treatment in the future. This will foreseeably allow his health system to save 600 lives in the future. However, the new treatments will take a long time to come online and will not benefit any of the identified persons currently suffering from AIDS. Without present treatment, these people will soon die.
> - *Prevention*: Spend all available funds on prevention, reducing the number of people in his district who will contract, and die from, AIDS in the future. This will foreseeably save 750 lives. However, again, without present treatment, the identified people currently suffering from AIDS will soon die.

I have argued, *pace* Brock and Wikler, that while prevention may maximize the number of lives saved, there is at least a pro tanto reason to choose present treatment instead, since this benefits the people who have the strongest claim on our assistance.

But what if, for some reason, Present Treatment is not an option, that is, we can choose only between Future Treatment and Prevention? In this case, Prevention appears both optimific and the option that would be favored by the ex ante view. For, in this case, the only people whose interests are at stake are people not yet suffering from AIDS. In other words, the only deaths we can prevent in this scenario are statistical deaths. In that case, it is in the ex ante interest of everyone concerned, that is, of anyone who is at some risk of contracting HIV/AIDS in the future, that we choose Prevention. For this is the option that most reduces everybody's risk of death ex ante. Choosing Prevention over Future Treatment, when these are our only two options, would therefore be unfair to no one.

A similar point can be made in response to the mining analogy that Brock and Wikler used to illustrate the supposed irrationality of privileging identified over statistical lives. ("No resources will be spared to try to rescue trapped miners . . . even if [less costly] safety measures that would have prevented the cave-in were deemed too expensive the previous year.") The behavior described here is irrational, even by the lights of the ex ante view. What we are dealing with is a choice, from the ex ante perspective, between two different methods of averting deaths from a future mining disaster: preventing the disaster by increasing safety, or waiting until a cave-in has occurred and then rescuing those trapped in the mine. Under these circumstances, it is obvious that we ought to choose the more cost-effective option, which is Prevention.

The AIDS pandemic, however, is different. Because it is an ongoing problem, our decision is never taken from a point of view that is ex ante for everyone. The mine accident, so to speak, has always already happened to some individuals, and we must decide how to respond: by rescuing those currently trapped in the mine and certain to die soon if we do not help them, or by "cutting our losses" and investing in future prevention. This, I have argued, is a harder moral problem, and one which a focus on individual claims and fairness can help to illuminate.

9. Postscript: Does "Treatment-as-Prevention" Transcend the Dichotomy between Treatment and Prevention?

One of the most exciting new avenues of AIDS research over the past few years revolves around the possibility of "treatment-as-prevention" (TasP). TasP is based on the hypothesis that starting HIV-positive patients on antiretroviral drugs at a very early stage of the disease can have significant preventive benefits for their sexual partners. The World Health Organization currently recommends that persons living with AIDS begin antiretroviral treatment when their CD4+ count (a measure of cells in the blood that reflect the status of the immune system) drops below 350. By contrast, a recent randomized control trial (HPTN 052) showed that initiating antiretroviral treatment at an earlier, largely asymptomatic stage of the disease (when the patient's CD4+ count is between 350 and 550) can reduce the risk of HIV-transmission to their HIV-negative partners by up to 96% (National Institute of Allergy and Infectious Diseases 2011). (For a helpful overview of the scientific, economic, and moral issues surrounding TasP, see the chapter by Till Bärnighausen and Max Essex, in this volume).

If the champions of TasP are right, the interests of people already suffering from AIDS in receiving treatment and the interests of the rest of the population in being protected from the disease may be more in alignment than my discussion has so far assumed. To a certain degree, treatment is prevention. All else equal, by treating current, identified sufferers of HIV/AIDS, we also reduce the number of statistical victims among their sexual partners and (via sexual transmission chains) in the population at large.

Despite its considerable scientific promise, however, I do not believe that TasP renders moot the ethical debate between proponents of treatment and of prevention that has occupied us in this chapter. Indeed, given limited health budgets in many of the countries worst affected by AIDS, there currently exist alternatives that are ethically preferable to TasP whichever side of the treatment versus prevention debate we stand on.

Consider, first, how things look from the perspective of the pluralist competing-claims view that I have advocated in this chapter. As Bärnighausen and Essex note, citing work by De Cock and El-Sadr (2013), there is still significant debate about whether receiving antiretroviral drugs at very early, asymptomatic disease stages has any significant medical benefit for the HIV-positive patient herself.[16] The primary rationale for initiating antiretroviral treatment at CD4+ levels above 350, therefore, is not its therapeutic effect for the infected patient but rather the preventive benefit for the patient's sexual partners (and their partners' partners, etc.).

Second, because of the high cost of TasP compared to conventional antiretroviral treatment, it is feared that rolling out TasP in many poorer countries would necessarily result in resources being reallocated from the treatment of some of the sickest HIV sufferers to the treatment of HIV-positive individuals at an earlier, asymptomatic disease stage (when the risk of transmission to sexual partners is arguably highest and TasP could have the biggest preventive

---

[16] Moreover, Kitahata et al. (2011) note possible undesirable side effects of early antiretroviral treatment, including diabetes, body fat changes, and—if treatment is not taken exactly as prescribed—an increased risk of drug resistance.

effect) (Haire 2011; Bärnighausen and Essex, this volume). In effect, we would treat fewer symptomatic patients overall, in order to start treating the patients we do treat sooner and thereby reap the preventive benefits of early antiretroviral therapy.

In resource-poor countries, moving from the present regime of antiretroviral therapy to a regime of TasP may thus require us to trade off the interests of some current symptomatic victims of HIV (whom we will no longer have the resources to treat if we implement TasP) against the interests of those at risk of becoming infected. This confronts policymakers with precisely the sort of moral issue that this chapter has attempted to illuminate. If, as I have argued, a policymaker has reasons of fairness to give somewhat greater weight to saving the lives of people who, but for her intervention, would be very likely to shortly die of HIV/AIDS rather than to further reduce other people's risk of contracting AIDS, this is a pro tanto consideration against cutting back on conventional antiretroviral therapy in favor of TasP or other preventive measures. So much is true at least in settings where limited resources do not permit all HIV-positive individuals to receive antiretroviral therapy at both early and advanced stages of the disease.

Suppose, however, that you disagree with my arguments in this chapter. Suppose you believe, like Brock and Wikler, that the only thing that matters morally in a choice between TasP and other methods of combating the AIDS pandemic is how many lives, or perhaps more precisely, how many QALYS, we can save with each method. In that case, too, you have reasons to be skeptical about TasP as the primary method for fighting AIDS in a resource-poor setting. Research by Bärnighausen and coauthors (2012) indicates that TasP is much less cost-effective, in terms of QALYs saved per dollar spent, than purely preventive interventions such as male medical circumcision. (Indeed, for the time being, it is less cost-effective even than conventional antiretroviral treatment limited to advanced stages of the disease.) Given this, choosing TasP over more cost-effective methods of prevention would, for an act-consequentialist, still show an objectionable bias toward helping identified victims over preventing statistical losses.

Proponents of rolling out TasP in resource-poor settings thus confront the following dilemma: either (1) it is morally justified to give some priority to saving identified victims at an elevated risk of death over preventing statistical losses. In that case, there is some reason to prefer conventional antiretroviral therapy to TasP, since this will allow the largest number of symptomatic patients to receive antiretroviral treatment. Or (2) there is no justification for giving priority to treatment over prevention; we ought simply to do what maximizes the number of QALYs we save. But in that case, too, TasP is bested by other, more cost-effective preventive interventions.

Hence, barring a dramatic fall in the cost of antiretroviral treatment, TasP cannot transcend the dichotomy between the objective of QALY maximization given to us by a pure consequentialist perspective and the stronger emphasis on fairness embodied by the competing claims model. The ethical debate between proponents of treatment versus prevention for HIV/AIDS, it seems, will remain a live one for the foreseeable future.

References

Bärnighausen, T., D. E. Bloom, et al. 2012. "Economics of Antiretroviral Treatment vs. Circumcision for HIV Prevention." *Proceedings of the National Academy of Sciences USA* 109 (52): 21271–76.
Brock, D., and D. Wikler. 2009. "Ethical Challenges in Long-Term Funding for HIV/AIDS." *Health Affairs* 28 (6): 1666–76.
Broome, J. 1990. "Fairness." *Proceedings of the Aristotelian Society* 91: 87–101.
———. 1994. "Fairness versus Doing the Most Good." *Hastings Center Report* 24 (4): 36–39.
Daniels, N. 2012. "Treatment and Prevention: What Do We Owe Each Other?" In *Prevention vs. Treatment: What's the Right Balance?* edited by H. Faust and P. Menzel, 176–93. Oxford: Oxford University Press.
De Cock, K. M., and W. M. El-Sadr. 2013. "When to Start ART in Africa: An Urgent Research Priority." *New England Journal of Medicine* 368 (10): 886–89.
Frick, J. 2013. "Uncertainty and Justifiability to Each Person: Response to Fleurbaey and Voorhoeve." In *Inequalities in Health: Concepts, Measures, and Ethics*, edited by N. Eyal, S. Hurst, O. Norheim, and D. Wikler, 129–46. New York: Oxford University Press.
———. n.d. "Contractualism and Social Risk: How to Count the Numbers without Aggregating." Manuscript.
Fried, C. 1969. "Value of Life." *Harvard Law Review* 82 (7): 1415–37.
Haire, B. 2011. "Treatment-as-Prevention Needs to Be Considered in the Just Allocation of HIV Drugs." *American Journal of Bioethics* 11 (12): 48–50.
Jenni, K., and G. Loewenstein. 1997. "Explaining the 'Identifiable Victim Effect.'" *Journal of Risk and Uncertainty* 14: 235–57.
Kamm, F. 1993. *Morality, Mortality.* Vol. 1: *Death and Whom to Save from It.* New York: Oxford University Press.
———. 2007. *Intricate Ethics.* Oxford: Oxford University Press.
———. 2009. "Aggregation, Allocating Scarce Resources, and the Disabled." *Social and Political Philosophy* 26: 148–97.
Kitahata, M., et al. 2011. "Effect of Early versus Deferred Antiretroviral Therapy for HIV on Survival." *New England Journal of Medicine* 360 (18): 1815–26.
Marseille, E., P. Hoffman, and J. Kahn. 2002. "HIV Prevention before HAART in Sub-Saharan Africa." *Lancet* 389: 1851–56.
Moore, R. 1996. "Caring for Identified versus Statistical Lives: An Evolutionary View of Medical Distributive Justice." *Ethology and Sociobiology* 17 (6): 379–401.
Nagel, T. 1991. *Equality and Partiality.* Oxford: Oxford University Press.
National Institute of Allergy and Infectious Diseases. 2011. "Treating HIV-Infected People with Antiretrovirals Protects Partners from Infection." NIH News, National Institutes of Health.
Rawls, J. 1999. *A Theory of Justice.* Rev. ed. Oxford: Oxford University Press.
Reibetanz Moreau, S. 1998. "Contractualism and Aggregation." *Ethics* 108: 296–311.

Scanlon, T. M. 1998. *What We Owe to Each Other*. Cambridge, MA: Harvard University Press.

Schelling, T. 1968. "The Life You Save May Be Your Own." In *Problems in Public Expenditure Analysis*, edited by S. Chase, 127–62. Washington, DC: Brookings Institute.

Taurek, J. 1977. "Should the Numbers Count?" *Philosophy & Public Affairs* 6 (4): 293–316

Temkin, L. 2012. *Rethinking the Good: Moral Ideals and the Nature of Practical Reasoning*. New York: Oxford University Press.

14 }

From Biology to Policy
ETHICAL AND ECONOMIC ISSUES IN HIV
TREATMENT-AS-PREVENTION

Till Bärnighausen and Max Essex

1. Background

1.1. A SHORT HISTORY OF HIV TREATMENT-AS-PREVENTION

HIV treatment has been one of the largest interventions in the history of public health. From 2000 until 2011 an estimated 8 million people were started on lifelong HIV antiretroviral treatment, the majority in sub-Saharan Africa (WHO 2011). The primary purpose of this global intervention has been to reduce mortality due to HIV (Mboup et al. 2006), as countries heavily affected by HIV experienced dramatic reversals of general worldwide trends of steadily increasing life expectancy over the past three decades (Bor et al. 2013).

While millions of people were initiated on antiretroviral therapy (ART) for their own health, research pointed toward a link between HIV viral load in blood and other body fluids and the likelihood of transmitting the virus during unprotected sex to others. It was hoped that ART could reduce the probability of HIV transmission in an unprotected sex act by lowering viral load (Quinn et al. 2000; Cohen et al. 2012). This research culminated in results from predictive mathematical models suggesting that large reductions in HIV incidence could be achieved if ART coverage of HIV-infected people reached very high levels (Granich et al. 2009; Eaton et al. 2012; Hontelez et al. 2013) and, more powerfully, the results of the HPTN 052 study establishing that early ART of the HIV-infected partner in a sero-discordant couple can nearly eliminate transmission to the HIV-uninfected partner (Cohen et al. 2011).

Since the results from the landmark HPTN 052 study have been published, several cluster-randomized controlled trials have been started to test the effectiveness of treatment-as-prevention in the general population of communities in sub-Saharan Africa with high HIV prevalence (Granich et al.

2010; Bärnighausen and Dabis 2013), including the Treatment-as-Prevention (TasP) ANRS 12249 trial in South Africa (Iwuji, Orne-Gliemann, et al. 2013); PopART HPTN 071 trial in South Africa and Zambia (HIV Prevention Trials Network 2014); and the Botswana Combination Prevention Project (BCPP) (Centers for Disease Control and Prevention 2013). In addition, a study of one of Africa's largest HIV incidence cohorts in rural South Africa, where ART is only provided in more advanced disease stages, found that an individual's risk of HIV infection decreased significantly with increasing ART coverage in the individual's local community (Tanser et al. 2013).

For the purpose of this chapter, we assume that we are in a world where it has been firmly established that HIV treatment can significantly reduce HIV incidence in general populations affected by the HIV epidemic. Here, we are concerned with the ethical and economic issues that will present themselves once treatment-as-prevention has been identified as effective in generalized HIV epidemics. In this chapter, we will discuss ethical and economic issues raised by treatment-as-prevention strategies, but we will not attempt to either discuss them exhaustively or to offer solutions or policy recommendations. We will also not discuss the differential ethical and economic issues that arise from particular approaches to HIV treatment-as-prevention, even though some aspects that distinguish alternative approaches may be ethically relevant, for instance, whether an approach will aim to initiate all HIV-infected individuals on ART or only those who fulfill additional viral load criteria (Novitsky and Essex 2012). Our goal is thus merely to raise awareness for ethical and economic issues, so that further debate and analysis can prepare us for a world where the effectiveness of HIV treatment-as-prevention in general populations has been firmly established and policies need to be designed.

1.2. TREATMENT-AS-TREATMENT VERSUS TREATMENT-AS-PREVENTION

ART can theoretically have three types of effects: (1) a treatment effect alone, (2) a prevention effect alone, and (3) both treatment and prevention effects. While in general ART will have both therapeutic and preventive effects, it will not have preventive effects in population groups who are not sexually active; and it is an ongoing debate whether HIV treatment in very early disease stages benefits the treated individual in Africa (De Cock and El-Sadr 2013), even though the US ART guidelines have recently recommended that all HIV-infected adults, irrespective of their disease stage and immunological functioning, should start HIV treatment (Thompson et al. 2012; Panel on Antiretroviral Guidelines for Adults and Adolescents 2013). These distinctions are important for the discussion of ethical and economic dimensions of HIV treatment-as-prevention policies. For instance, the ethical permissibility of HIV treatment-as-prevention recommendations will vary depending on whether treatment will always or only sometimes have beneficial effects for the treated person's own health. When taking ART is the best strategy for improving one's own health, questions of the ethical permissibility of motivating people to start HIV treatment for preventive purposes are far less complex, since they do not need to involve considerations of the trade-off between a person's own well-being and the health of others.

A further important consideration for the discussion of ethical issues in HIV treatment-as-prevention is that, as a general rule, the mortality benefits of ART increase as HIV disease advances. Similarly, the preventive effect of ART is likely to increase with HIV disease progression because in advanced disease stages the viral load, and thus HIV transmission probability per unprotected sex act, is higher than in earlier stages (with the exception of a short period immediately after HIV infection). However, since HIV transmission is a function of both the rate of unprotected sex acts and the transmission probability per act, the preventive effect gradient with disease stage is far less certain than the therapeutic effect gradient. After all, it is plausible that sicker people have less sex or use condoms more frequently than healthier people, which could result in a larger preventive effect of ART in earlier compared to later stages of HIV disease. In this chapter, we will either refer to "HIV treatment-as-prevention" strategies as ART strategies with the *primary purpose* of preventing HIV (rather than prolonging the lives of HIV-infected people) or we will precisely describe to which combination of ART prevention and treatment effects we are referring.

2. Issues in HIV Treatment-as-Prevention

2.1. ALLOCATING RESOURCES TO POLICIES

While it is likely that HIV-infected persons in all disease stages derive some benefit from ART for their own health, it is also well established that the health benefits in advanced disease stages, in particular mortality reductions, are larger than those in early disease stages. Furthermore, when there are binding HIV budget constraints, interventions other than ART, most notably male medical circumcision, "compete" for resources as opportunities to avoid health loss through HIV treatment or prevention. As a recent economic evaluation of combinations of HIV interventions shows, HIV treatment-as-prevention is highly cost-effective but far less cost-effective (both in terms of averting new infections and saving lives) than either ART constrained to those in late disease stages or male medical circumcision (Bärnighausen, Bloom, et al. 2012). According to these results, to attain the utilitarian objective of minimizing health losses given constrained resources, HIV treatment-as-prevention should only be implemented once coverage with male medical circumcision and ART for those in late disease stages have reached universal or near-universal levels.

2.2. POLICIES WITHOUT RESOURCES FOR ALL

Currently, to receive ART in a sub-Saharan African country, an HIV-infected person needs to have reached advanced disease stages, which are operationalized through CD4 cell counts capturing immunological functioning and clinical staging based on physical examination and past medical history. Treatment-as-prevention strategies would open up formal eligibility to receive ART to people in less advanced disease stages. In countries where resource constraints preclude the provision of ART to all those who are eligible under current guidelines, treatment-as-prevention strategies could conceivably lead to "crowding out of ART" of people who are sicker by those who are less sick (Bärnighausen et al. 2014). For instance, it is plausible that healthier people will be able to demand the treatment they are formally eligible to receive more vigorously and more often than sicker people. Such a "crowding out" would violate most nonutilitarian consequentialist and nonconsequentialist conceptions of fairness in access to healthcare. It is thus unlikely that treatment-as-prevention strategies are intended to produce "crowding out"; it is much more likely an unintended consequence that has so far not been considered in discussions of treatment-as-prevention for some of the poorest countries in the world. A policy option avoiding this consequence is to enlarge the pool of people eligible for ART to include those in early disease stages for treatment-as-prevention only if lifelong treatment for both those in early and all those in late disease stages can be guaranteed.

2.3. MOTIVATING UPTAKE

The effectiveness of treatment-as-prevention strategies will depend on high levels of uptake of HIV treatment by individuals in early disease stages. Currently, people expressing demand for ART in sub-Saharan Africa are on average in relatively advanced disease stages—more advanced than the disease stages at which people first become eligible to receive ART under the current guidelines. It is thus likely that the main motivating factor for people to seek treatment is HIV symptoms (which are rare in most early disease stages) rather than motivations that are also likely to be present in early disease stages, such as wanting to find out about one's health or psychological anxiety (Bärnighausen, Salomon, et al. 2012; Bärnighausen and Dabis 2013). The fact that the typical person who is currently on ART started utilizing the treatment in comparatively advanced disease stages does not imply that "crowding out" described above will not occur under treatment-as-prevention strategies. For "crowding out" to occur and cause ethical worry, it is sufficient that some people in early disease stages demand treatment and are provided treatment instead of some people who are in more advanced disease stages. Treatment-as-prevention strategies, however, usually assume that large proportions of people in early disease stages need to receive ART.

This requirement then raises the question which additional interventions are ethically permissible to motivate the uptake of ART in early disease stages. While the current policy debates seem to assume that demand for ART can be substantially increased by expanding HIV counselling and testing (HCT) coverage, HCT interventions alone are unlikely to lead to substantial increases in demand for ART. In settings such as South Africa, where knowledge of both HIV status and HIV in general is high, ART coverage has not been more vigorous than in many other settings where HIV knowledge is far poorer (WHO 2011); and in most settings large proportions of people who know that they are HIV-positive have never accessed HIV clinical services (UNAIDS 2011; Bärnighausen and Dabis 2013). Additional interventions may thus be necessary to ensure the success of treatment-as-prevention strategies, and many candidate interventions may be opposed on ethical grounds. Coercive measures are usually considered unjustifiable as general public health policies (Annas 2007), including for preventing the transmission of diseases that unlike HIV have very high mortality rates despite optimal treatment, such as extremely drug-resistant tuberculosis (South African Medical Research Council 2007). Financial incentives may be seen as unduly inducing treatment uptake; and social pressure may be feared to increase HIV-related stigma and to harm already vulnerable populations. Perhaps the ethically most appealing approach is information campaigns targeted at HIV-infected populations, which explain that taking antiretroviral drugs can protect transmission of the virus to loved ones (Vandormael et al. 2014). However, such campaigns may not be sufficiently effective to ensure that the full population health impact of HIV treatment-as-prevention is realized.

HIV treatment-as-prevention has added a powerful argument for increasing ART utilization. Ethical debate will be necessary to determine how far the preventive effects of ART lead to a normative obligation of HIV-infected individuals to take ART, even if they would not (yet) be motivated to do so for their own health and well-being, and how far such an obligation could justify strong persuasion, material incentives, or penalties to motivate ART uptake.

2.4. IDENTIFIED VICTIM EFFECTS AND HIV TREATMENT-AS-PREVENTION

Identified victim effects refer to the tendency of people to express greater willingness to alleviate the suffering of identified individuals as compared to "statistical" persons who are not individually known but merely characterized by their potential to benefit from an intervention (Jenni and Loewenstein 1997; Kogut and Ritov 2005). In the history of HIV in the United States, the passage of the Ryan White Care Act has been attributed to an identified victim effect. The suffering and death of Ryan White, one particular, publicly identified HIV patient who contracted HIV following treatment for his hemophilia, is thought to have influenced the passage of the act carrying his name more than the abstract suffering expressed in HIV disease statistics (Reagan 1990).

For HIV treatment-as-prevention, identified victim effects may play out differently at different levels of decision-making. At the policy level, the potential victims at risk of contracting HIV are statistical persons. By definition of the prevention of a probabilistic event, the future victims of the HIV epidemic are not yet identifiable with certainty when decisions about prevention interventions are made. It may be possible to describe the characteristics of persons at comparatively high risk of acquiring HIV, but the concrete persons contracting HIV in the future are unknown. In contrast, for the individual HIV-infected person deciding whether to take up HIV treatment and prevention, the immediate potential victims who can benefit from his intervention uptake are clearly identified and emotionally immediate: the sex partners in unprotected sex acts. At the individual level, the preventive nature of the intervention does not imply unidentifiability; the event, HIV transmission, is probabilistic but the initial beneficiary of the reduced transmission probability is known and the emotional attitudes of the decision-maker to the person will usually be highly positive. The case becomes more complex when we consider "victims" in the broader sexual networks of the decision-maker. Along sexual HIV transmission chains, identifiability will be reduced with distance from the decision-maker (the sex partners of one's sex partner, the sex partners of one's sex partner's sex partners, and so on). The emotional attitudes towards these "victims" will vary depending on the precise circumstances of partnership formation; they may be highly negative (e.g., jealousy) or positive (a feeling of solidarity, for instance, among members of a group with a particular sexual orientation).

Identified victim effects have commonly been thought of as biases, moving decisions away from the normatively right decision. Indeed, identified victim effects are often called identified victim biases. The bias is usually viewed as a deviation from a utilitarian objective, such as minimizing health loss—we are saving fewer identified lives rather than more statistical ones (Fried 1969). If identifiable victim effects are indeed biases, we do not have to worry about them distorting decisions on HIV treatment-as-prevention. At the policy level, the potential victims are unidentifiable; at the individual level the first-order effects, people's inclinations to preferentially act to protect identified persons to whom they feel emotionally attached, will improve the uptake and thus the success of treatment-as-prevention as they will counteract the general tendency of HIV-infected people in sub-Saharan Africa to seek healthcare only in late stages of HIV disease.

2.5. IDENTIFIED VICTIM EFFECTS AND HIV TREATMENT VERSUS PREVENTION

If, however, the identified victim effect is not a bias leading to normatively wrong decisions, the case becomes more complicated. Consequentialist objections against the claim that the tendency to save fewer identified rather than more statistical lives is normatively wrong include redefinitions of the objective (McKie and Richardson 2003; Daniels 2012)—for example, minimizing health loss and maximizing the joy derived that someone else's health loss has been reduced instead of merely minimizing health loss—and arguments that reducing the health loss of an identified rather than a statistical victim will lead to lower health losses in the long run because the identification with the victim motivates future health loss-reducing action (Small et al. 2007). Norman Daniels discusses these and nonconsequentialist objections against the claim that identified victim biases lead to normatively wrong decisions. He concludes that reasonable people disagree on this question because of a "lack of consensus on principles that resolve the disagreement" (Daniels 2012, 43).

If identified victim effects are not biases leading to normatively wrong decisions, there are two possible cases regarding what "statistical victim effects" represent. In the first case, the distribution of identifiability across different victims is such that the influences of both identified and statistical victim effects will lead to the normatively right decision. It seems unlikely, however, that the distribution of identifiability should always be "right" because it is unstable and will change frequently due to the influences of many factors that are at least partially determined by chance, such as media reports, the existence of a particular technology that can be used to visualize the suffering of some types of victims, the occurrence of a disease in a family that is willing and able to present the suffering of a family member to the public, and so on. It would seem an odd concept if chance decided between what is normatively right and wrong.

In the second case, decisions will be normatively wrong without the correcting influence of an identified victim effect. David Canning has argued that one reason for the substantially higher investment in HIV treatment than in HIV prevention, despite the higher cost-effectiveness of prevention, could have been the individual identifiability of the people currently suffering from advanced HIV disease and the unidentifiability of those who in the future might contract HIV (Canning 2006). If we accept that the identifiability of people currently suffering from HIV disease has led to a normatively right level of investment in HIV treatment, it might be the case that HIV prevention efforts have remained underfunded relative to the normatively desirable levels. In this case, it would be the responsibility of decision-makers to seek out information or to engage in thought experiments to increase the identifiability of the victims of future HIV infection, in order to counteract the effects of a statistical victim bias on decision-making.

This second case would have implications for HIV treatment-as-prevention. The investment in treatment with the primary purpose of avoiding the health losses of the person already infected with HIV would not have deviated from the normatively right level because the victims are identifiable, but the future additional investments in treatment with the primary purpose of prevention are likely to remain underfunded. To move closer to the normatively desirable funding levels, the decision-makers would need to make the unidentified victims more identified, for instance, by envisioning the as-of-yet unknown people who will contract HIV as similar to those persons who are suffering from the disease today.

3. Conclusion

The potential to achieve large reductions in HIV incidence through treatment-as-prevention raises a number of ethical and economic issues, which have implications for policy and practice. What is the optimal resource allocation across different HIV treatment and prevention interventions, when treatment also functions as a preventive measure? How can we avoid the danger that HIV treatment-as-prevention policies lead to healthier patients crowding sicker patients out of treatment? What interventions are ethically permissible to motivate individuals who do not feel sick and may not yet benefit from ART to enroll in treatment for HIV prevention? Will identified victim effects distort resource allocation to HIV treatment-as-prevention away from the normatively desirable levels, and should we counteract such tendencies? The debate on HIV treatment-as-prevention has been largely focused on effectiveness. While the current evidence strongly suggests that ART prevents HIV transmission, the results of several large trials of different treatment-as-prevention strategies in some of the communities most severely affected by the HIV epidemic are still outstanding. The period spent waiting for the trial results offers an opportunity to resolve some of the ethical and economic questions raised by the potential to prevent HIV through treatment.

References

Annas, G. J. 2007. "Your Liberty or Your Life: Talking Point on Public Health versus Civil Liberties." *EMBO Reports* 8 (12): 1093–98.

Bärnighausen, T., and F. Dabis. 2013. "Implementation of HIV Treatment-as-Prevention: Resources and Behaviors." In *HIV Prevention*, edited by M. L. Newell and F. Tanser, 89–102. London: Future Medicine.

Bärnighausen, T., D. E. Bloom, et al. 2012. "Economics of Antiretroviral Treatment vs. Circumcision for HIV Prevention." *Proceedings of the National Academy of Sciences USA* 109 (52): 21271–76.

Bärnighausen, T., D. E. Bloom, et al. 2014. "Human Resources for Treating HIV/AIDS: Are the Preventive Effects of Antiretroviral Treatment a Game Changer?" Submitted.

Bärnighausen, T., J. A. Salomon, et al. 2012. "HIV Treatment as Prevention: Issues in Economic Evaluation." *PLoS Medicine* 9 (7): e1001263.

Bor, J., A. J. Herbst, et al. 2013. "Increases in Adult Life Expectancy in Rural South Africa: Valuing the Scale-Up of HIV Treatment." *Science* 339 (6122): 961–65.

Canning, D. 2006. "The Economics of HIV/AIDS in Low-Income Countries: The Case for Prevention." *Journal of Economic Perspectives* 20 (3): 121–42.

Centers for Disease Control and Prevention. 2013. "Botswana Combination Prevention Project (BCPP)." Available from http://clinicaltrials.gov/ct2/show/record/NCT01965470.

Cohen, M. S., Y. Q. Chen, et al. 2011. "Prevention of HIV-1 Infection with Early Antiretroviral Therapy." *New England Journal of Medicine* 365 (6): 493–505.

Cohen, M. S., C. Holmes, et al. 2012. "HIV Treatment as Prevention: How Scientific Discovery Occurred and Translated Rapidly into Policy for the Global Response." *Health Affairs (Millwood)* 31 (7): 1439–49.

Daniels, N. 2012. "Reasonable Disagreement about Identified vs. Statistical Victims." *Hastings Center Report* 42 (1): 35–45.

De Cock, K. M., and W. M. El-Sadr. 2013. "When to Start ART in Africa: An Urgent Research Priority." *New England Journal of Medicine* 368 (10): 886–89.

Eaton, J. W., L. F. Johnson, et al. 2012. "HIV Treatment as Prevention: Systematic Comparison of Mathematical Models of the Potential Impact of Antiretroviral Therapy on HIV Incidence in South Africa." *PLoS Medicine* 9 (7): e1001245.

Fried, C. 1969. "Value of Life." *Harvard Law Review* 82 (7): 1415–37.

Granich, R., S. Crowley, et al. 2010. "Highly Active Antiretroviral Treatment as Prevention of HIV Transmission: Review of Scientific Evidence and Update." *Current Opinion in HIV and AIDS* 5 (4): 298–304.

Granich, R. M., C. F. Gilks, et al. 2009. "Universal Voluntary HIV Testing with Immediate Antiretroviral Therapy as a Strategy for Elimination of HIV Transmission: A Mathematical Model." *Lancet* 373 (9657): 48–57.

HIV Prevention Trials Network. 2014. "Population Effects of Antiretroviral Therapy to Reduce HIV Transmission (PopART)—NCT01900977." Available from http://clinicaltrials.gov/ct2/show/NCT01900977.

Hontelez, J. A., M. N. Lurie, et al. 2013. "Elimination of HIV in South Africa through Expanded Access to Antiretroviral Therapy: A Model Comparison Study." *PLoS Medicine* 10 (10): e1001534.

Iwuji, C. C., J. Orne-Gliemann, et al. (2013). "Evaluation of the Impact of Immediate versus WHO Recommendations-Guided Antiretroviral Therapy Initiation on HIV Incidence: The ANRS 12249 TasP (Treatment as Prevention) Trial in Hlabisa Sub-district, KwaZulu-Natal, South Africa: Study Protocol for a Cluster Randomised Controlled Trial." *Trials* 14: 230.

Jenni, K. E., and G. Loewenstein. 1997. "Explaining the 'Identifiable Victim.'" *Journal of Risk and Uncertainty* 14 (3): 235–57.

Kogut, T., and I. Ritov. 2005. "The 'Identified Victim' Effect: An Identified Group, or Just a Single Individual?" *Journal of Behavioral Decision Making* 18: 157–67.

Mboup, S., R. Musonda, et al. 2006. "HIV/AIDS." In *Disease and Mortality in Sub-Saharan Africa*, 2d ed., edited by D. T. Jamison, R. G. Feachem, et al., 237–46. Washington, DC: World Bank.

McKie, J., and J. Richardson. 2003. "The Rule of Rescue." *Social Science and Medicine* 56 (12): 2407–19.

Novitsky, V., and M. Essex. 2012. "Using HIV Viral Load to Guide Treatment-for-Prevention Interventions." *Current Opinion on HIV and AIDS* 7 (2): 117–24.

Panel on Antiretroviral Guidelines for Adults and Adolescents. 2013. *Guidelines for the Use of Antiretroviral Agents in HIV-1-Infected Adults and Adolescents*. Washington, DC: Department of Health and Human Services.

Quinn, T. C., M. J. Wawer, et al. 2000. "Viral Load and Heterosexual Transmission of Human Immunodeficiency Virus Type 1: Rakai Project Study Group." *New England Journal of Medicine* 342 (13): 921–29.

Reagan, R. 1990. "We Owe It to Ryan." *Washington Post*, January 11.

Small, D., G. Loewenstein, et al. 2007. "Sympathy and Callousness: The Impact of Deliberative Thought on Donations to Identifiable and Statistical Victims." *Organizational Behavior and Human Decision Processes* 102: 143–53.

South African Medical Research Council. 2007. "Detention of Patients with Extensively Drug-Resistant Tuberculosis (XDR-TB)." Available from http://www.mrc.ac.za/pressreleases/2007/1pres2007.htm.

Tanser, F., T. Bärnighausen, et al. 2013. "High Coverage of ART Associated with Decline in Risk of HIV Acquisition in Rural KwaZulu-Natal, South Africa." *Science* 339 (6122): 966–71.

Thompson, M. A., J. A. Aberg, et al. 2012. "Antiretroviral Treatment of Adult HIV Infection: 2012 Recommendations of the International Antiviral Society-USA panel." *JAMA* 308 (4): 387–402.

UN Programme on AIDS (UNAIDS). 2011. *Global HIV/AIDS Response: Epidemic Update and Health Sector Progress towards Universal Access*. Geneva: UNAIDS.

Vandormael, A., M. L. Newell, et al. 2014. "Use of Antiretroviral Therapy in Households and Risk of HIV Acquisition in Rural KwaZulu-Natal, South Africa, 2004-12: A Prospective Cohort Study." *Lancet Global Health* 2 (4): e209–e215.

World Health Organization (WHO). 2011. *Towards Universal Access: Scaling Up Priority HIV/AIDS Interventions in the Health Sector*. Geneva: WHO.

15 }

Testing, Treating, and Trusting

Jonathan Wolff

Deciding how to spend limited funds on HIV measures throws up a difficult dilemma for those who control budgets. People who are already HIV-positive and are suffering from the symptoms of AIDS can be provided with medication that in the best cases turns a life-threatening infection into a controllable chronic condition. Unfortunately, however, treatment is typically very expensive to administer, even if the cost of many drugs has fallen dramatically. Alternatively, money could be spent on preventative measures such as condom distribution, male circumcision, and education. It is sometimes argued that if our concern is to get the greatest health benefit for our money, preventative measures are to be preferred, as they can save many more lives for the same expenditure (Cohen, Neumann, and Weinstein 2008). Condom distribution, for example, is very cheap, and if it directly prevents even one HIV infection, then indirectly it may prevent very many over time, as there will be one fewer infected person to infect others. Hence a DALY-minimizing (or QALY-maximizing) HIV strategy could possibly entail devoting perhaps the entire HIV budget to prevention, saving many more (statistical) lives (Charania et al. 2011). Yet if you were the budget allocator, in a district where individuals with developed AIDS symptoms were not receiving the treatment that could be funded within your budget, what would you do? Could you really ignore the person in front of you, who has severe symptoms that will end his or her life very soon, but could at some expense be treated so that he or she is returned to something close to a normal life? Or would you nevertheless hold firm in deference to cost-effectiveness arguments and devote the budget to prevention, thereby saving the most statistical lives? Few of us, I believe, would be prepared to go the whole way with the consequentialist maximizing reasoning that mandates spending it all on prevention. Hence, it seems, helping identified people has a very strong moral pull on us, even if less good overall will be done that way. Hence, the moral dilemma of whether to give priority to fewer identified lives over more statistical ones is felt acutely in HIV policy.

The idea of "treatment as prevention," however, holds out at least a glimmer of hope that the dilemma can be transcended.[1] Suppose it turns out that treatment is an effective preventative strategy. In that case one can engage in both prevention and treatment through the same means: the provision of treatment. No decision needs to be made about whether to treat identified or statistical lives, as both happen at once. Now, whether this really solves the dilemma depends on a number of factors. For example, if treatment is a very expensive form of prevention, then consequentialism will still mandate other, cheaper approaches, which will do more good for the same amount of money. There is, then, an empirical question about costs and benefits, and it may well be that the calculation still comes out against the treatment as prevention. Yet on some assumptions the calculation will be favorable. Modern triple therapy will very often reduce an individual's viral load to the point where he or she is barely infectious. One recent study shows almost miraculous results. In the experimental arm of the study, in which early therapy was offered, there was only one transmission from an HIV-positive person to his or her previously uninfected partner; in the control arm, involving standard, delayed therapy, there were twenty-seven (Cohen et al. 2011). Of course, on its own this tells us little about the cost-effectiveness of rolling out an entire program, but it does at least provide a starting point.

The immediate lesson from this study appears exceptionally encouraging: it is possible to imagine mathematical models in which the epidemic is entirely eliminated in just a few generations. If so, and if we can design policies that can implement the mathematical models, there is an argument that we ought to scale up treatment hugely. Even if it costs a vast amount of money in the short and medium term, the long-term saving if the epidemic disappears would be immense. Treating the current (identified) generation saves huge numbers of (statistical) future individuals. Elimination is the ultimate prevention and over enough time will be more cost-effective than strategies that do not eliminate the problem (ignoring discount rates). These, at least, are the appearances. Yet we also know that appearances can be deceptive.

First, we need to keep in mind that the study referred to above was a very unusual one. It was a study of people in stable relationships, which raises a number of issues. For one, these people are probably not in the highest-risk groups. For another, someone in a stable relationship probably has a very strong emotional attachment to his or her partner, which will influence behavior, particularly in terms of feeling responsibility to another person when it comes to ensuring that medication is being taken. These facts may present

---

[1] For doubts, however, see the earlier chapters in this part of the book.

some obstacles for implementing treatment as prevention on a larger scale, especially when it includes, as it must, individuals who do not have such settled lives.

Treatment as prevention is also known as "Test and Treat." There are issues of concern around both the testing side of this strategy and the treatment side. On the testing side, if elimination is the goal, then every infected person has to be brought within the treatment program, and thus every infected person needs to be tested early on. Currently this does not happen, and the prospects are not encouraging. In the current state of the world, it is not always irrational to remain untested even if you are worried about your HIV status. There have been times when the level of stigma that one still finds in parts of Africa has caused people who are HIV-positive to be ostracized by their families, beaten, attacked, and even murdered (Nolen 2007). And there are areas in the world with close and tightly knit communities where it is not easy to keep secrets, so that the best way to avoid declaring your status as HIV-positive is not finding out yourself. There is, then, a huge barrier to voluntary testing in many parts of the world. If individuals do not come forward for testing, then they may well infect others, and there is nothing treatment as prevention can do about this. Before we can roll out anything like Test and Treat on the scale needed to make major inroads into the epidemic, there has to be another type of work that has to happen in order to address the stigma of living with HIV. (Of course, there are independent reasons for wanting to perform this work anyway.)

So the testing side will not be straightforward. What about the treatment side? Here my point is best made by engaging in a detour. Consider something that may seem very different: road safety. In a study in the United Kingdom, Dr. Ian Walker and colleagues cycled around Bristol sometimes wearing a helmet, sometimes without a helmet, and sometimes wearing a long blond wig. When the cyclist wore a helmet cars drove closer to the bike; when the cyclist wore a long blond wig and no helmet, cars kept a little further away (Walker 2007). Presumably motorists thought that a cyclist wearing a helmet is more likely to ride in a competent fashion and so needs less margin for error. This is one of many possible illustrations of the claim that others will adjust their behavior to take into account their beliefs about how safe or unsafe the actions of others are. If someone does not seem to pose a threat, then others need to take fewer precautions. A reputation for safety can lead others to relax. Therefore, an undeserved reputation for safety can be very dangerous.

How does this bear on Test and Treat? Recall that under conditions such as the one in the study cited above, involving stable couples, the person receiving treatment was presumably highly compliant with treatment. That person would have been perceived as safe, and correctly so. But imagine someone who has a more casual sexual life. This potential partner tells you that you do not need to worry about other forms of HIV protection because he is on the Test and Treat regime. Do you believe him?

Consider an analogy. Suppose there were a male contraceptive pill that was just like the female contraceptive pill and has to be taken every day. Imagine it does not have serious side effects, but like any pill is something of a nuisance to take. Those taking it have to remember to take it every day, and to remember to renew their prescriptions. Would such a pill catch on? In fact, people are generally not very good at complying with medical treatment, especially when they do not feel the immediate benefit. For instance, it is well known that one of the reasons drug-resistant tuberculosis has developed is that patients often fail to complete their drug treatments because they stop when they feel better, even though they need to continue taking drugs for the course of treatment to be effective. This is why DOT (directly observed therapy) was introduced (Pablos-Mendes et al. 1997).

It is, of course, not the case that people never take their medications. For those who have suffered serious symptoms of AIDS, begun triple therapy and experienced the so-called "Lazarus" effect of recovery, there is every reason to continue treatment with great resolution. A memory of how bad things were can assist continued adherence to treatment. But taking medication under other circumstances—in this case essentially for altruistic reasons—is likely to be much more problematic from the point of view of compliance. How problematic this turns out to be will partly depend on what precise level of compliance to the treatment is sufficient to keep the risk of infection very low. If it is perfectly okay to miss a month, then the problem is reduced. But if viral load rises whenever medication use is irregular, then treatment will fail to be preventative. And unlike the case of condom use, a sexual partner is unable to check whether preventative measures have been taken. Hence, Test and Treat critically involves trust, and if that trust is misplaced, then a belief in safety may lead couples to neglect other preventative strategies, at great cost.

Accordingly, just as it is perfectly conceivable that allowing a male contraceptive pill onto the market would actually increase the amount of unplanned pregnancies by allowing a new form of deception and complacency, it is perfectly conceivable that rolling out treatment as prevention at a very large scale would actually increase the rate of HIV transmission. The danger is that people would be less prone to engage in other needed preventative techniques because of their (false) perceptions of their sexual partner's compliance.

Perhaps, however, we could try to incentivize people to do the right thing by providing additional rewards or payment for compliance. There is some evidence that this can work, although unfortunately there are few examples of successful incentivizing that results in continued good behavior even when incentives are taken away (Marteau, Ashcroft, and Oliver 2009). More promising, however, are cases where we have seen voluntary behavior change involving people coming to recognize that they are imposing risks on third parties. Arguably, smoking in the United

Kingdom, for instance, fell more rapidly when smokers began to consider the harm they were imposing on other people; for then they started to feel bad about the way they were behaving (alternative explanations, such as the indignant response of those who regard themselves as harmed, may also be possible). Quite possibly when smokers thought they were only harming themselves, smoking bans were thought of as annoying governmental interference in private lives.[2] But one thing to keep in mind here is that the people who present the highest risk (the most adamant smokers, say) may very well be the least concerned about the risk they impose on others. Many people still smoke. In the context of Test and Treat, it not unreasonable to speculate that the people who engage in the riskiest sexual behavior are also likely to be the most causal about regularly taking their medication.

Sadly, treatment as prevention on its own will not end the HIV epidemic (and thereby transcend the dilemma of whether to save identified or statistical lives). It could only do so if everyone who was HIV-positive came forward for early testing, and then was fully compliant with treatment for the rest of his or her life. In the absence of assurance on both of those points, it is one preventative strategy among others, and like other preventative strategies, before it is rolled out on a large and costly scale to the potential detriment of other preventative strategies, we should consider the settings in which it will and will not work. It may be particularly beneficial for sero-discordant couples who wish to have children and therefore do not want to use condoms, as well as for others who live settled lives in stable relationships. On a broader scale, however, a widespread belief that infection has been controlled by treatment could be very dangerous.

In conclusion, while it remains true that treating the identified person in front of you has the very welcome effect of reducing that person's viral load and thus making him or her less infectious, and thus posing less of a threat to (at this point) statistical others, unfortunately the moral dilemma remains. Although early testing and treatment of an HIV-positive person will both aid an identified person and help save statistical lives (assuming that the medication is kept up), it is very likely that the same money spent on condom distribution will do much more good as a preventative strategy. Test and treat, though it prevents HIV, does not prevent hard choices about which programs to support.

Acknowledgments

I would like to thank members of the audience at the Harvard Global Health Institute Conference on Identified versus Statistical Lives 2012, as well as the

---

[2] Perhaps regulators hoped for this kind of effect when on UK television and at cinemas they embarked on an advertising campaign that showed a teenage boy in the back seat of the car not wearing a seatbelt, who in an accident flew forward and killed his mother in the driver's seat. For one response to the smoking ban, see the artist David Hockney's thoughts (Hockney 2007).

Institute for help with writing up these remarks and Norman Daniels and Nir Eyal for their very helpful comments on an earlier draft, as well as those of an anonymous referee.

References

Charania, Mahnaz R., Nicole Crepaz, Carolyn Guenther-Gray, Kirk Henny, Adrian Liau, Leigh A. Willis, and Cynthia M. Lyles. 2011. "Efficacy of Structural-Level Condom Distribution Interventions: A Meta-analysis of U.S. and International Studies, 1998–2007." *AIDS Behavior* 15: 1283–97.

Cohen, Joshua T., Peter J. Neumann, and Milton C. Weinstein. 2008. "Does Preventive Care Save Money? Health Economics and the Presidential Candidates." *New England Journal of Medicine* 358: 661–63.

Cohen, M. S., Y. Q. Chen, et al. 2011. "Prevention of HIV-1 Infection with Early Antiretroviral Therapy." *New England Journal of Medicine* 365: 493–505.

Hockney, David. 2007. "I Smoke for My Mental Health." *The Guardian*. Available from http://www.theguardian.com/artanddesign/2007/may/15/art.smoking.

Marteau, T., R. Ashcroft, and A. J. Oliver. 2009. "Using Financial Incentives to Achieve Healthy Behaviour." *British Medical Journal* 338: 983–85.

Nolen, Stephanie. 2007. *28 Stories of AIDS in Africa*. New York: Walker.

Pablos-Méndez A., C. A. Knirsch, R. G. Barr, B. H. Lerner, and T. R. Frieden. 1997. "Non-adherence in Tuberculosis Treatment: Predictors and Consequences in New York City." *American Journal of Medicine* 102 (2): 164–70.

Walker, Ian. 2007. "Drivers Overtaking Bicyclists: Objective Data on the Effects of Riding Position, Helmet Use, Vehicle Types and Apparent Gender." *Accident Analysis and Prevention* 39: 417–25.

INDEX

Abbott Laboratories v. Gardner, 169
aboriginal islanders, 78, 89
abortions, 165
act-consequentialism
    interpersonal aggregation and, 185
    Life versus Headaches case and, 190
    Mass Vaccination case and, 193–95
acute care interventions, 49
Adamson, Harry, 83n7
Adler, Matthew, 5–6, 64n13, 80n5
advisory opinions, 162
affect heuristic, 26–27, 36
affective primacy, 27
Africa, 203–4, 206–8, 215
agent-relative prerogatives, 78n1, 117–18, 120
aggregate litigation, 170
aggregation, 3, 5–6, 79, 118, 142–43
    antiaggregationist principles, 7, 131–35
    benefits and, 46–47
    cost-effectiveness and, 46
    interpersonal, 185, 188
AIDS. *See* HIV/AIDS
air pollution, 2, 175
air travel, 142–43, 142n3
Allen, Woody, 85
analysis. *See also* cost-benefit analysis
    axiomatic, 63
    thinking conditions, 17
The Anatomy of Values (Fried), 153
Andaman Islands, 78, 89
animals, 4
    dual-process model and, 28–31
    endangered, 19
    Endangered Species Act, 164
Anonymity, 63
anonymous victims, 19
Anthony, Casey, 13
Anthony, Caylee, 13
antiaggregationist principles, 7, 131–35
antiretroviral therapy (ART), 9, 182–83, 187, 198–200, 199n16, 203–7
anxiety, 58
ART. *See* antiretroviral therapy
Ashford, Elizabeth, 142–43
Asian tsunami, 20
asthma, 161, 166, 174, 179

attunement, 30
axiomatic analysis, 63

babies, 31
bad effects, distribution of, 7, 132–33
Bank Secrecy Act, 168
Bärnighausen, Till, 9, 199
Battle of Britain, 6, 102
Bayesian learning, 31–33
BCPP. *See* Botswana Combination Prevention Project
benefits, 25. *See also* cost-benefit analysis
    aggregation and, 46–47
    cost-effectiveness and, 49
    forward models of, 31
    health, 49, 213
    interpersonal aggregation and, 185
    magnitude of, 35–36
    probability of, 34–35
    regulatory, 179
    urgency and, 45
Benjamin Braddock (fictional character), 85
best outcomes/fair chances problem, 119
bias, 1–4, 19
    applications of, 8–10
    consequentialism and, 113–15
    distributional equity and, 130–31
    ethics and political philosophy and, 5–8
    HIV/AIDS and, 208–9
    merely statistical people and, 125–30
    nonconsequentialism and, 116–20
    social science and, 4–5
    sources of, 111
    of sympathy, 20
bioethics, 125, 184, 197
birds, food-caching, 29–30
Botswana Combination Prevention Project (BCPP), 204
Bovens, L., 66n16
Brady, James, 13
Brady Handgun Violence Prevention Act, 13
brain-imaging studies, 31
Brock, Dan W., 5, 182–85, 196, 198
bronchitis, 174, 179
Broome, John, 97
"bucket list" expenditures, 60n11
Burson, K. A., 19

219

Calabresi, Guido, 113
California Bankers Association v. Shultz, 168
cancer, 19, 175, 179
    of Chamberlain, 97–98
    drugs and, 2
    pollution and, 174
Canning, David, 209
catastrophe-averse, 64n13
caudate, 30
causal connection, 156
causal immediacy, 157
Caylee's Law, 13
CBA. *See* cost-benefit analysis
certainty
    risk and, 87–88
    of threat, 111
    uncertainty, 5, 48–49, 57, 66–69
certification, 170–71
ceteris paribus PSIV, 54–55, 57–59, 60n11, 62, 68
Chamberlain, Neville, 97–99, 106
charitable donations, 114
charities, 129n6
Chemerinksy, Erwin, 162
children, 155
    asthma and, 161, 166
    babies, 31
Chilean mining accident, 1, 144
choice simulators, 37
chronic diseases, 20
Churchill, Winston, 94–95, 97, 99–102, 101n5, 104–5, 104n7
circumcision, medical, 205–6, 213
City of Los Angeles v. Lyons, 163–64
civil litigation, 8, 161–62
    class actions and, 170–72
    conclusion to, 172
    justiciability and, 162–70
    representative victim and, 170–72
    standing and, 162, 163–66
class actions, 170–72
Clean Air Act, 2, 175–76
coal burning, 161
Cohen, Glenn, 8, 126n3, 129n7, 151, 154–56
Cohen, Josh, 120
coherent grouping, 19
coin flipping, 100, 119, 127–28
collectivism, 7
    RoR and, 139, 144–48
commonality prerequisite, 171
communication, 32
community, 145–47, 146n5
compensating variation, 70
competing claims, 185–88, 195
complaint model, 186
concentrated risk. *See* risk concentration

concrete examples, 111
concrete facts, 168
condom distribution, 213
congenital heart surgeries, 3
congenital metabolic diseases, 137
consequentialism, 8, 110, 209
    act-consequentialism, 185, 190, 193–95
    ex ante Pigou-Dalton principle and, 68, 69*t*
    in favor of bias, 113–15
    nonconsequentialism and, 110, 116–20
    objections to bias, 113
    PSIV and, 56, 64–66, 65*t*, 66n16
    special relationships and, 50
    SWF and, 55n3, 66, 74–75
constant marginal disvalue claim, 91
Constitution, US, 162, 166, 170
constitutive compactness, 157
constitutive solidarity, 145–46
contraception, 165, 216
contractualism, 7, 139–41, 148
    demandingness of, 142–43
    risk aversion and, 142–43
controlled experiments, 15
Copiapó, Chile mining accident, 1, 144
cost-benefit analysis (CBA), 5, 54n2, 55n3, 56, 59–62, 67*t*, 178
    monetary equivalents and, 58n7
    PSIV and, 71–73
    risk-cost-benefit analysis, 115
    Risk Transfer and, 71–73
    VSL and, 70–71
cost-effectiveness, 2–3
    aggregation and, 46
    benefits and, 49
    equal concern and, 101
    HIV/AIDS and, 9–10, 182, 200, 205, 209, 214
    mining accidents and, 1, 144, 147
    RoR and, 137–39, 146–47, 148
    temporal discounting and, 49
counterfactual conditionals, 84–85
counterfactual indeterminacy, 124–25
    antiaggregationist principles and, 7, 131–35
    conclusion to, 135
    distributional equity and, 130–31
    statistical people and, 125–30
Court of Appeals, First Circuit, 167
Coventry Blitz attack, 94–97, 94n1, 99–102, 101n5, 104–6
Craig v. Boren, 166
Crime Victims' Rights Act, 180
crowding out, 206
curative treatment, 138

Daley, William, 177
Daniels, Norman, 6–7, 9, 156–57, 187, 209

concentrated risk and, 95–97
distributional equity and, 130–31
equal concern and, 100–101
"dead anyway" effect, 60
death permutation, 64–65, 64n14
decision theorists, 184
De Cock, K. M., 199
Deepwater Horizon oil rig, 174
Defenders of Wildlife, 164
dehumanization, 114–15
Delaware, 171
demandingness, of contractualism, 142–43
democratic processes, 121
deontology, 55, 103, 152
Departments of Interior and Commerce, 164
descriptive projects, 25
deterministic laws, 127
dialysis, 2
dictator game, 15
diffusion, 157
disasters, 20. *See also specific disasters*
diseases, 2. *See also* cancer; HIV/AIDS
  chronic, 20
  congenital metabolic, 137
  epizootic, 142–43
  fundraising for, 44
  infectious, 140
  lysosomal storage, 137
distributional equity, 130–31
distributive fairness, 97, 106
Doe v. Bolton, 165
drinking age, 166
dual-process models, 4, 16–17, 25–28
  animals and, 28–31
  asymmetry of, 24–25
  implicit social competence and, 33–36
  looking forward and, 36–38
  magnitude of benefit or harm and, 35–36
  probability of benefit or harm and, 34–35
  System 1 and, 31–33
  System 2 and, 31–33
Dworkinians, 99

earthquakes
  in Haiti, 13
  in Japan, 13, 20
easy rescues, 115
economist's strategy, 113
effectiveness, 29. *See also* cost-effectiveness
efficiency, 29
emergency rooms, 45
emotional thinking conditions, 17
emotion-based motivation, 151
emotions, 8, 150–51
empathy, 26, 116, 150–57

causal connection and, 156
development of, 155
partiality and, 153–54
psychology and, 152–53
second-order chill, 154–55
endangered animals, 19
Endangered Species Act, 164
Enigma cipher, 94, 94n1
environmental issues, 49
environmental law, 8–9, 161, 174–80
Environmental Protection Agency (EPA),
  175–77, 179–80
enzyme replacement therapy, 137
EPA. *See* Environmental Protection Agency
epistemic improbability, 81
epistemic probability, 80
epistemic risks, 77–78, 80
  concentration of, 99, 101, 103
  interpretations of, 98
  pooling, 102–3
epistemology, 25
epizootic diseases, 142–43
equal concern, 99–102
equality, social, 99
Equal Protection Clause, 166
equity, 56, 66–69
  distributional, 130–31
  equity-regarding SWFs, 63–66, 67t
equivalent variation, 70
Ernst & Young v. Depositors Economic
  Protection Corp., 167
Essex, Max, 9, 199
ethical rationalism, 151
ethics, 5–8, 24–25. *See also specific topics*
  bioethics, 125, 184, 197
  virtue, 8
evenly weighted, 128
evolutionary theory, 35
ex ante, 5–7, 48
  equity-regarding SWF, 67t
  evaluation, 111–12
  HIV/AIDS, view of, 190–91
  leximin, 66, 68
  methodologies, 56
  Pareto principle, 68, 69t
  Pigou-Dalton principle, 54n2, 56, 65–66,
    68, 69t
  SWF, 56, 63–64, 64t
  utilitarianism, 56, 67t, 74–75
expectation-based models, 31, 33
expectation formation, 34
expected value, 27, 33
experimental studies, 26
ex post, 5–7, 48
  equity-regarding SWF, 56, 67t

Index } 221

ex post (*Cont.*)
  evaluation, 111–12
  HIV/AIDS, view of, 190–94
  methodologies, 56
  RoR and, 141–44
  SWF, 56, 63–64, 64t
  utilitarianism, 56, 67t
externalities, 113, 114
extremist morality, 116
Eyal, Nir, 5, 6, 119n2

fairness, 56, 195–96
  distributive, 97, 106
  in health care access, 206
Faro, D., 19
Farrow, Mia, 85
fatality risk, 59–60
favoritism, 99–100
FDA. *See* Food and Drug Administration
fear, 58
Federal Poverty Level (FPL), 46
feedback, 32
First Circuit Court of Appeals, 167
fitness criterion, 167
fixed budget, of health expenditures, 138
Fleurbaey, M., 66n16
Food and Drug Administration (FDA), 169
food-caching birds, 29–30
Food Quality Protection Act, 175
forward models, 31, 34
FPL. *See* Federal Poverty Level
Frederick, S., 16
Frick, Johann, 6, 9, 95, 97, 104n7, 118n1, 119n2
Fried, Charles, 1, 113, 115, 117, 153–54
friendship, 19, 117
From Enlightenment to Receptivity: Rethinking Our Values, 155
fully equalized cases, 117
fundraisers, 2, 44
future possibilities, mental simulation of, 26

Gaddafi, Muammar, 177
Galak, J., 16
gender bias, 114–15
Gibbard, Allan, 114–15
Glover, Jonathan, 105–7
good effects, concentration of, 7, 133
government intervention, 54
The Graduate (film), 85
greater obligations, 126
Griswold v. Connecticut, 165

Habitat for Humanity, 15, 24, 34
Haidt, Jonathan, 28
Haiti earthquake, 13

Hájek, Alan, 132n12
Hamlet (fictional character), 85
Hammitt, J. K., 64n13
hardship claims, 167, 168
Hare, Caspar, 6–7, 119n2
harm
  discounting, 77–92
  magnitude of, 35–36
  probability of, 34–35
Harvard University, 150, 156
HCT. *See* HIV counselling and testing
health
  ART and, 203, 205
  benefits, 49, 213
  environmental law and, 8–9, 174–75, 177, 180
  expenditures, 138
  policy, 21, 25, 33, 37, 207
  prioritization, 45–46
  professionals, 37–38
  PSIV and, 54
  public, 9
health care, 2–3
  decision-making in, 37
  fairness in access to, 206
  policy, 29, 37–38
  politics of, 24
  priority to the worse off and, 47
  public, 137, 147–48
  RoR and, 137
  urgency and, 45
heart attacks, 79, 174
heart surgeries, congenital, 3
Heinzerling, Lisa, 8–9
heuristics, 32, 37
  affect, 26–27, 36
  simulation, 36
hippocampus, 30
HIV/AIDS, 20, 51
  Brock and, 182–85
  competing claims and, 185–88
  cost-effectiveness and, 9–10, 182, 200, 205, 209, 214
  ex ante view of, 190–91
  ex post view of, 190–94
  pluralist account of moral rightness and, 194–96
  pro identified lives argument and, 188–90
  resource allocation and, 4, 199, 205–6, 210
  RoR and, 184
  temporal structure and, 196–98
  Test and Treat for, 213–17
  treatment-as-prevention and, 198–201, 203–10
  Wikler and, 182–85

HIV counselling and testing (HCT), 207
Hoffman, Dustin, 85
Holloway, Natalee, 13
homelessness, 20
Hsee, C. K., 27
Hume, David, 116, 153–54
Hurricane Katrina, 20

identified lives, 5–6, 43–44, 50–51, 110–13, 114
  aggregation and, 46–47
  CBA and, 56, 62
  civil litigation and, 161–72
  environmental law and, 8–9, 174, 176–77
  ethics and political philosophy and, 5–6
  HIV/AIDS and, 9, 182, 185–88, 196–97
  priority to the worse off and, 47–48
  Pro Identified Lives Argument, 188–90
  RoR and, 44–45
  special relationships and, 50
  standing and, 163, 165–66
  temporal discounting and, 49
  uncertainty and, 48–49
  urgency and, 45–46
  welfarism and, 56
Immigration and Naturalization Service (INS), 169
implicit social competence, 33–36
  magnitude of benefit or harm and, 35–36
  probability of benefit or harm and, 34–35
implicit stereotyping, 37
improbability, epistemic, 81
incoherent grouping, 19
income
  Risk Transfer and, 61
  status quo, 60–61
indirectness, 157
individualism, 139
infectious diseases, 140
injury-in-fact jurisprudence, 163, 170
INS. *See* Immigration and Naturalization Service
interpersonal aggregation, 185, 188
interpretations of risk, 98
Intricate Ethics (Kamm), 196n15
intrinsic moral value, 43
intuitionism, 151
intuitive decision-making, 16–17, 24, 27–28
intuitive sense, 36
Ipilimumab (drug), 2

Jackson, Lisa, 176
Japan earthquake, 13, 20
Jenni, Karen E., 111–12, 117, 156, 157
Jones, B., 18
Jonsen, Albert, 1, 44, 137

judicial restraint, 166
justiciability
  ripeness and, 162, 166–70
  standing and, 162, 163–66
justification, 139

Kagan, Shelly, 116
Kahneman, Daniel, 16, 28, 31, 36, 121
Kamm, Frances, 117, 119–20, 151, 187n7, 196n15
Kant, Immanuel, 151–52
Katrina (hurricane), 20
kidnap victims, 14
kidney failure, 2
kin-selection theory, 18
kinship, 117
Kirlin, Dennis M., 171
Kitahata, M., 199n16
Kiva.org, 16
Kogut, T., 15, 26, 35
Korsgaard, Christine, 151
Kripke, Saul, 152, 154

language, 32
large-scale disasters, 20
law. *See also* civil litigation
  aggregate litigation, 170
  Caylee's Law, 13
  deterministic, 127
  environmental, 8–9, 161, 174–80
  sham litigation, 162
Lazarus effect of recovery, 216
lesser obligations, 126
Lewis, David, 127n4
leximin, 66, 68
Libya, 177
Life versus Headaches case, 185–86, 190, 196n15
The Limits of Kindness (Cohen, G.), 126n3, 129n7
linguistic intuitions, 32
livestock farming, 142–43
Loewenstein, George, 111–12, 117, 156–57
  affect heuristic and, 26–27
  charitable donations and, 114
  controlled experiments by, 15
  victim statistics and, 17
lottery, 106–7, 132–33
Lujan v. Defenders of Wildlife, 164
Lyons, Adolph, 163–64
lysosomal storage diseases, 137

male medical circumcision, 205–6, 213
mammals, 29
marginal disvalue claim, 91
margin of safety, 175

Mass Vaccination case, 192–95, 193n10
mathematical models, predictive, 203
maximization arguments, 10
maximizing strategy, 113
McClure, Jessica, 110, 176
McKie, John, 114
media, 13, 112, 125, 144, 209
Medicaid, 46
medical circumcision, 205–6, 213
Medicare, 2
melanoma, 2
merely statistical people, 125–30
metabolic diseases, congenital, 137
metaphysics, of open counterfactuals, 84–85
microfinance, 16
Milgram experiments, 18
mining accidents, 145–47, 146n5, 153–55, 184, 198
  in Copiapó, Chile, 1, 144
models. *See also* dual-process models
  complaint, 186
  expectation-based, 31, 33
  forward, 31, 34
  predictive mathematical, 203
  weather, 129n6
monetary equivalents, 58n7, 59–60
Monty Hall problem, 32
mootness, 162
moral deliberation, 139–40
moral obligations, 124–25
moral rationalism, 151
moral rightness, 186
  pluralist account of, 194–96
moral sentimentalism, 8, 151–52, 154–55
Moral Sentimentalism (Cohen, G.), 151, 154, 156
moral value, 43–44
mortality matrix, 59, 59t, 65t
motivation, emotion-based, 151
multiprocess theories, 16–17

naming, 156
Naming and Necessity (Kripke), 152
National Ambient Air Quality Standards, 2, 175
national support, 147
nearness, 117, 120
neurological deficits, 174
neurology, 30
neuroscience, 28
neutrality, 113
nonconsequentialism, 110
  in favor of bias, 116–20
  objections to bias, 116
nonepistemic risks, 99
  concentration of, 104–7
  interpretations of, 98
normative enterprises, 25

normative theory, 14
nuclear waste, 49

Obama, Barack, 37, 176–77
objective probability, 80n5
objective risks, 83, 83n7
obligations
  greater, 126
  lesser, 126
  moral, 124–25
Occupational Safety and Health Act (OSHA), 175
Office of Information and Regulatory Affairs (OIRA), 178–79
Office of Policy (EPA), 179
Ohio, 168
oil spill, Deepwater Horizon, 174
OIRA. *See* Office of Information and Regulatory Affairs
"one thought too many" case (Williams), 152
One versus Eight case, 189
One versus 50 case, 189, 190, 195–96
One versus Five case, 190–91, 195
One versus One case, 187, 188–89, 191
open counterfactuals, 126–29
  metaphysics of, 84–85
Oregon, 46
organ transplantation, 46
OSHA. *See* Occupational Safety and Health Act
Otsuka, Michael, 5, 6, 95, 97, 101, 119n2
ozone, 177–78

Pareto principle, 63
  ex ante, 68, 69t
Parfit, Derek, 49
partiality, 102, 153–54
peer monitoring, 16
peer screening, 16
permanent scarcity, 45
persistent scarcity, 45–46
person-affecting antiaggregationist principle, 7, 131–35
personalists, 117
pesticides, 175
physical probability, 80n5
Pigou-Dalton principle, 63
  ex ante, 54n2, 56, 65–66, 68, 69t
Pinera, Sebastian, 1
pluralism, of moral rightness, 194–96
Policymaker's Trilemma case, 197
political philosophy, 5–8
political theory, 125
pollution, 2, 161, 174–80
PopART HPTN 071 trial, 204
post hoc rationalizations, 28
poverty, 16, 20

predators, 29
predictive mathematical models, 203
presidential elections, 37
preteens, 155
preventive interventions, 183
prey, 29
Principle of the Equal Moral Worth of All Human Lives, 43, 49, 50
prioritarian SWFs, 63
prioritization, 141
  health, 45–46
  resource allocation and, 47
Priority for Saving Identified Victims (PSIV), 53–55
  CBA and, 71–73
  ceteris paribus, 54–55, 57–59, 60n11, 62, 68
  consequentialism and, 56, 64–66, 65t, 66n16
  risk permutation and, 73–74
  Risk Transfer and, 61, 73–74
priority to the worse off, 5, 47–48
probability, 6, 31, 57
  of benefit or harm, 34–35
  epistemic, 80
  epistemic improbability, 81
  interpretations of, 98
  matching, 32
  objective, 80n5
  physical, 80n5
  statistical, 80n5
procedural justice, 121
procrastination, 184
Pro Identified Lives Argument, 188–90
PSIV. *See* Priority for Saving Identified Victims
psychological distancing, 4, 17–19
psychological numbing, 14
psychology, 13–14, 28
  conclusion to, 20–21
  empathy and, 152–53
  empirical evidence in lab and field, 14–16
  mechanisms for preference, 16–19
  RoR and, 44–45
public health care, 137, 147–48
public policy, 120–21
The Purple Rose of Cairo (film), 85
push-button emotional responses, 28, 37

quality-adjusted life year (QALY), 2, 3, 185n5, 200

Rachlin, H., 18
racism, 99, 100, 114–15
Railton, Peter, 4
Ramsey, JonBenet, 13
Rapoport, Anatol, 105
rationalism, 8
  ethical, 151

Kantian, 152
  moral, 151
rational solidarity, 145–46
rational strategy, 113
rats, 30
Rawls, John, 120, 186
Reagan, Ronald, 13, 178
realized goodness of lives, 58
real time, 111
reasonable disagreement, 120–21
"Reasonable Disagreement about Identified vs. Statistical Victims" (Daniels), 156
reattunement, 30
red fix, 152, 154
redressability, 163n2
reference-dependent sympathy, 20
reference groups, 14, 111–12
regulatory benefits, 179
Reibetanz Moreau, Sophia, 78n1, 87–88, 191
REM sleep, 30
Reno v. Catholic Social Services, 169
representative life, 162
representative victim, 170–72
reproductive abnormalities, 174
resource allocation, 19, 29, 143
  HIV/AIDS and, 4, 199, 205–6, 210
  prioritization and, 47
  in public health care, 147–48
  RoR and, 138, 144
  to TasP policies, 205–6
  timing of, 144
  utilitarianism and, 14, 21
rhetorics, 147
Richardson, Jeff, 114
ripeness, 162, 166–70
risk, 3, 58
  aversion, 48, 142–43
  certainty and, 87–88
  distribution of, 103, 107
  epistemic, 77–78, 80, 98–99, 101–3
  fatality, 59–60
  interpretations of, 98
  nonepistemic, 98–99, 104–7
  objective, 83, 83n7
  reduction, 62
  social, 192, 194
risk concentration, 96–97, 102–4, 112, 118–20
  conclusion to, 107
  epistemic, 99, 101, 103
  equal concern and, 99–102
  meaning of, 97–99
  nonepistemic, 104–7
risk-cost-benefit analysis, 115
risk permutation, 66, 66n15
  Risk Transfer and, 73–74

risk pooling, 95, 99, 103
risk seeking with regard to losses, 112
Risk Transfer, 54, 61, 66
  CBA and, 71–73
  risk permutation and, 73–74
Ritov, I., 15, 26, 35, 36
RoR. *See* rule of rescue
Rottenstreich, Y., 27
rule of rescue (RoR), 1, 5, 7, 114
  collectivist argument for, 144–48
  collectivist perspectives of, 139
  conclusion to, 148
  cost-effectiveness and, 137–39, 146–47, 148
  ex post perspectives of, 141–44
  HIV/AIDS and, 184
  individualist perspectives of, 139
  psychology and, 44–45
  sympathy and, 138
  what we owe to individual patients, 139–41
rules of thumb, 32
Russian roulette, 82–84, 82n6
Ryan White Care Act, 208

Sacrifice Known Limb, 77–81
Sacrifice Unknown Life (dust), 77–81, 82–84, 87, 89, 92
Sacrifice Unknown Life (wheel), 81–85, 87–89, 92
Sacrifice Unknown Number of Lives (guns), 85–86, 89, 92
El-Sadr, W. M., 199
safety regulations, 54
same number non-identity case, 125
Savage, Leonard, 57
Scanlon, Tim, 7, 148, 151, 187n7
  aggregation and, 142–43
  justification and, 139
  World Cup case of, 80
Schelling, Thomas, 1, 14, 113, 125n2, 183n1
Schkade, D., 36
second-order empathic chill, 154–55
self-conscious deliberation, 34
sentimentalism, 8, 151–52, 154, 155
separateness of persons, 186
sham litigation, 162
Sher, George, 97, 101
simulation heuristic, 36
Singer, Peter, 8, 117, 153
Slote, Michael, 6, 8
Slovic, Paul, 17, 26, 27, 114
Small, Deborah A., 4, 15–17, 26–27, 111, 114
Smith, R. W., 19
smoking, 216–17
social competence, implicit, 33–36
social equality, 99
Socialist Labor Party v. Gilligan, 168

social risk, 192, 194
social science, 4–5, 125
social utility theory, 17
social value, 44
social welfare function (SWF), 54n2, 56, 59, 62–66
  consequentialism and, 55n3, 66, 74–75
  equity-regarding, 63–66, 67t
  ex ante, 56, 63–64, 64t
  ex post, 56, 63–64, 64t
  prioritarian, 63
  utilitarian, 63–64
  well-being and, 56
solidarity, 7, 145–48, 146n5
  constitutive, 145–46
  rational, 145–46
South Africa, 204, 207
special relationships, 5, 50
Stalin, Joseph, 3, 91
Stalnaker, Robert, 127n4
standing, 162, 163–66
  third-party, 165–66
state courts, 170
states of the world, 57
statistical lives, 1, 19–20, 43–44, 50–51, 110–13
  aggregation and, 46–47
  civil litigation and, 161–72
  environmental law and, 8–9, 174–80
  ethics and political philosophy and, 5–6
  HIV/AIDS and, 9, 182–83, 185–88, 191, 196–97
  personalists and, 117
  priority to the worse off and, 47–48
  Pro Identified Lives Argument and, 188–90
  psychological distancing and, 19
  RoR and, 44–45
  special relationships and, 50
  temporal discounting and, 49
  uncertainty and, 48–49
  urgency and, 45–46
  welfarism and, 56
statistical probability, 80n5
status quo, 53, 57, 70
  income, 60–61
Stephen, A., 16
stereotyping, implicit, 37
stimulus-triggered motor habits, 30
strictly rational budget, 115
studies
  brain-imaging, 31
  experimental, 26
suboptimal giving, 19
sub-Saharan Africa, 203, 206, 208

Sunstein, Cass, 178
supervenience, 55n3
Supreme Court, 162–65, 163n2, 167–68, 170–71. *See also specific cases*
SWF. *See* social welfare function
symbolic value, 113, 115
sympathy, 4, 13–16, 19, 26, 116
  reference-dependent, 20
  RoR and, 138
System 1 (intuitive and emotional system), 16–17, 27–28, 29, 31–33
System 2 (deliberate system), 17, 28, 31–33

TasP. *See* treatment-as-prevention
Taurek, John, 187n7
teenagers, 155
temporal discounting, 5, 49
temporal structure, 196–98
temporary scarcity, 45
Test and Treat, 213–17
Thinking, Fast and Slow (Kahneman), 28
third-party standing, 165–66
time depth, 33
time horizons, 29, 33
T-mazes, 30
Toilet Goods Association, Inc. v. Gardner, 169
traceability, 163n2
Treatise of Human Nature (Hume), 153, 154
treatment-as-prevention (TasP), 4, 9–10, 182, 198–201, 203–10, 214
  conclusion to, 210
  history of, 203–4
  identified victim effects and, 207–10
  issues in, 205–10
  resource allocation to policies, 205–6
  treatment-as-treatment versus, 204–5
  uptake and, 206–7
treatment-as-treatment, 204–5
Treich, N., 64n13
tsunami, Asian, 20
tuberculosis, 207
Tversky, Amos, 31, 121

UK. *See* United Kingdom
uncertainty, 5, 48–49, 57, 66–69
United Kingdom (UK), 2, 215–17
United States (US)
  air pollution in, 2, 175
  ART in, 204
  civil litigation in, 8, 161–72
  Constitution of, 162, 166, 170
  Deepwater Horizon oil rig and, 174
  Delaware, 171
  HIV/AIDS in, 207–8
  Ohio, 168

Oregon, 46
VSL and, 62
urgency, 5, 45–46
US. *See* United States
utilitarianism, 14, 21, 56, 67t, 139, 154
utilitarian SWFs, 63–64
utility gap, 65

vaccinations, 118–19, 129–30, 140
  Mass Vaccination case, 192–95, 193n10
  risk concentration and, 96
  temporal discounting and, 49
value
  constant marginal disvalue claim, 91
  expected value, 27, 33
  moral, 43–44
  social, 44
  symbolic, 113, 115
value of statistical life (VSL), 59–60, 62, 70–71
vectors, 62–63, 65
Verweij, Marcel, 6, 7
victimhood, 19
victim statistics, 17
virtue ethics, 8
visual images, 111
vividness, of identification, 111–12, 156
Voorhoeve, Alex, 100n4
VSL. *See* value of statistical life

Walker, Ian, 215
Wal-Mart Stores, Inc. v. Dukes, 171
Wasserman, David, 100, 101
Water Supply case, 192–95, 193n10
weather models, 129n6
welfarism, 5, 54, 55–56, 55n3, 58. *See also* social welfare function
well-being, 58n8, 58n9, 61, 129n6
  fair distribution of, 55–56, 63
  realized goodness of lives and, 58
  supervenience and, 55n3
  SWF and, 56
western scrub-jays, 29–30
White, Ryan, 208
WHO. *See* World Health Organization
Wiggins, David, 152
Wikler, Daniel, 182–85, 196, 198
Williams, Bernard, 152
Wilmington Firefighters Local 1590 v. City of Wilmington, 171
Wolff, Jonathan, 10
World Cup case, 79–80
World Health Organization (WHO), 199
worse off, priority to, 5, 47–48

Zambia, 204

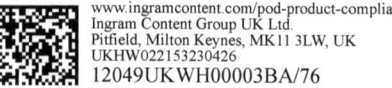
www.ingramcontent.com/pod-product-compliance
Ingram Content Group UK Ltd.
Pitfield, Milton Keynes, MK11 3LW, UK
UKHW022153230426
12049UKWH00003BA/76